OCR

D0909791

Choosing Medical Care
in Old Age

❖

CHOOSING MEDICAL CARE IN OLD AGE

❖ *What Kind* ❖

❖ *How Much* ❖

❖ *When to Stop* ❖

MURIEL R. GILLICK

Harvard University Press

Cambridge, Massachusetts

London, England

To Larry

❖

First Harvard University Press paperback edition, 1996

Text design by Gwen Frankfeldt in Adobe Minion

Library of Congress Cataloging-in-Publication Data

Gillick, Muriel R., 1951–
Choosing medical care in old age : what kind, how much,
when to stop / Muriel R. Gillick.
p.   cm.
Includes bibliographical references and index.
ISBN 0-674-12812-5 (cloth)
ISBN 0-674-12813-3 (pbk.)
1. Aged—Medical care.   I. Title.
RC952.G54   1994
362.1'9897—dc20

94-11333
CIP

❖ *Contents* ❖

Contents

❖ *Preface* ❖

This book has been five years in gestation. It was first conceived when I became convinced that if only the general public saw what I saw every day—what happened to older people when they became ill—there would be far more agreement than currently exists about what constitutes a reasonable approach to providing medical care for the elderly. In today's climate, the prevailing belief is that decisions about which of several alternative treatments to use, how much care to give, and when to stop are largely value decisions, based on the patient's preferences. In our pluralistic society, it is taken as a given that consensus on such a delicate matter as limitation of care is virtually impossible. It seemed to me that the situation was not exclusively a matter of individual preference: I felt that although there would always be a domain in which individuals could and should exercise choice based on their own beliefs, there was a much larger territory in which we could achieve agreement on the most appropriate strategy. The agreement, however, would arise not from a debate about ethical principles, but rather from a shared understanding of what is entailed by being old and sick.

When Daniel Callahan wrote his controversial book about limiting medical care to individuals on the basis of age, *Setting Limits,* I was even more determined to introduce the substance of real clinical cases into the debate over how best to approach medical care of the elderly. I agreed with Callahan that undesirable, inappropriate medical care was being inflicted upon millions of older patients, but I disagreed that the basis for limitation of medical treatment should be an age cutoff. The more patients I took care of—and I am a practicing internist who specializes in the elderly—the more convinced I became that I wanted to share their stories, indeed felt obligated to share their stories, in the hope that this would help forge a consensus about a reasonable overall approach to providing medical care for the growing elderly population. At the very least, the stories and surrounding commentary might help individuals faced with decision making for themselves or older relatives find some answers to the difficult questions concerning intensity of care.

I would not have embarked on this project without the many patients in whose anguish, sickness, and healing I was privileged to participate. The stories here are composites, based on the experience of many patients. In each case there is a core patient, a single individual whose tale forms the kernel of what I relate. For the preservation of confidentiality, names and other technical details have been modified. I have drawn on the biographies and clinical histories of other kindred patients to amplify my account. When I did not know certain facts about the lives of the patients, I felt free to embellish the narrative, seeking always to remain true to the character and circumstances of the core patient.

A number of people were particularly helpful to me in the creation of this book. Helen Epstein, Terri Fried, Martha Montello, and Robert Truog read parts of the manuscript and made invaluable suggestions. Edvardas Kaminskas and Lewis Lipsitz at the Hebrew Rehabilitation Center for Aged granted me a sufficiently flexible schedule to give me time to write. My editor at Harvard University Press, Angela von der Lippe, had the faith in me and in the spirit behind this book that I needed to persevere in my writing. Above all, my husband, Larry, has served as midwife to the project— checking up on my progress and encouraging me as I went along, and ultimately functioning as a calm but determined labor coach when the time came actually to produce the book.

My three children, Daniel, Jeremy, and Jonathan, managed to feel more pride than jealousy toward the book, even though they had to forgo many a game of Scrabble or Ping-Pong because I wanted to work instead of play. My parents, Ilse and Hans Garfunkel, aided and abetted the project both concretely, by helping to take care of my boys, and spiritually, through their boundless confidence in me.

❖ *Prologue* ❖

When I was midway through writing this book, my 81-year-old father-in-law developed a volvulus, a twist in the bowel. It was several days before the diagnosis was established, during which time he languished in the hospital, unable to eat or drink. He grew progressively weaker and ultimately required abdominal surgery to remove most of his large intestine. Although, in surgical jargon, he tolerated the operation well—meaning he did not have a heart attack or develop an infection or have massive bleeding—he took a long time to recover. It was a week before his intestines began to work and he could eat again. Once he resumed eating, he began having problems with explosive, unpredictable diarrhea. By the time he was discharged and returned home, a month after his initial bout of vomiting and abdominal pain, he was wobbly on his feet, he had lost fifteen pounds, and he was a bit disoriented, having been out of touch with the outside world for so long. Above all, he was extremely discouraged. Before his illness he had been independent and reasonably active. He had been accustomed to chauffeuring his wife around, had done the grocery shopping himself, and had vacuumed and dusted the apartment. Never before had he needed help with dressing or bathing. He had never in his adult life had to worry about getting to the bathroom in time. He felt, looked, and acted like an old man.

My father-in-law gradually improved. It was several months before his various physical problems sorted themselves out, and with the progress in walking and continence came an improvement in his spirits. Though he was significantly better, he never returned to his previous level of functioning. I was personally reminded of what I as a physician specializing in the care of the elderly knew professionally: the inevitability of at least sporadic illness, and in many cases of gradual decline, in older people. I was also struck by how utterly unprepared my in-laws were to face any major medical problems. They had not given any thought to how they would get along if one of them became ill. My mother-in-law had not kept up her driving skills and had become increasingly dependent on her husband for getting around, which presented a major dilemma when he became ill. Neither of them had designated a health care proxy, someone who would be legally empowered to make decisions for them if they were unable to speak for themselves—the issue had never come up. The two of them had vaguely considered the possibility that they might someday be unable to live fully independently in their current apartment. They were aware that some people join life care communities, in which they typically pay a sizable entrance fee to move into an apartment on a veritable senior citizen campus. Such communities usually provide meals in a communal dining room and supply modest assistance with personal care if necessary. Often a nursing home is available on the premises for either short-term rehabilitation after hospitalization or long-term care. They knew about other apartment complexes that offered "assisted living," on-site help with housekeeping and with personal care. But they had not actually visited such places nor even sent for literature, since no one had encouraged them to do so. My in-laws had never considered purchasing long-term care insurance to cover home care or nursing home care. They had always assumed that Medicare plus their savings would take care of all their needs, and no one had ever suggested otherwise.

Two months after my father-in-law was discharged from the hospital, my mother-in-law began developing pain in her side. She was a vigorous woman who looked ten years younger than she actually was. She led an active social life and had no medical problems other than mildly elevated blood pressure, for which she took one pill a day. In addition to the side pain, my mother-in-law suffered from headaches and noticed that she seemed to have lost her normally exuberant appetite. She assumed her headaches were due to the stress of taking care of her husband. She regarded the side pain as another minor inconvenience, attributing it to a pulled muscle, perhaps sustained while washing the countless loads of laundry generated during the course of her husband's illness. The weight loss was also easy to explain. Throughout the month when she had made daily trips to the hospital to visit her husband, she had often skipped a meal and skimped on the ones she did have. It seemed hardly worthwhile cooking for one person, so she had often just heated up a can of soup or poured a bowl of cereal. My mother-in-law's doctor was not convinced. He ordered a computerized tomogram (CT) scan. The scan showed that she had metastatic cancer throughout her abdomen.

My in-laws' world was shattered. Not only were they stunned by the news, they were also unprepared for the decisions they were suddenly asked to make. Should my mother-in-law consider chemotherapy? What if it made her sick? What if chemotherapy offered her a fifty percent chance of slightly prolonging her life—would she want it then? What if it offered only a twenty percent chance? How much of her remaining time was she willing to spend in a hospital? At what point would she accept hospice care, palliative care whose goal is maximization of comfort rather than prolongation of life? And who would take care of my father-in-law, who was no longer able to manage on his own, when his wife, his primary caretaker, herself became incapacitated, as she undoubtedly would?

I did not expect my in-laws to have figured out the answers to all these difficult questions in advance. In fact, I did not want them to have considered in excruciatingly painful detail the full range of unpleasant contingencies they might have to face. But I did wish I had prepared them for the fact that one day they would become sick; that they might well recover, but they would probably develop disabilities at some point, necessitating outside help; and that eventually they would die. I wished I had helped them discuss the general outlines of the kind of care they would want in each of several broad categories of situations in which they might find themselves. It pained me to see that they were living one day at a time, not daring to think about next week or next month, and certainly not about next year. They did this partly out of fear and denial, but largely I think because they had no framework in which to think about the decisions they might be called upon to make about their lives in general and their medical care in particular.

My in-laws are unusual in that they sustained two major blows to their health in a very short period of time. They began as a vigorous couple who took daily walks, who frequently visited friends and relatives, and who depended only on each other. They were excellent examples of what I as a geriatrician call the robust elderly. They had had a few medical problems over the years: he had very high blood pressure for which he took several medications; she had a history of slightly elevated blood pressure and took one medication. He had had bowel surgery some twenty years earlier; she had had cataracts removed from both eyes and wore contact lenses. Neither of them had had any problems that interfered with their activities of daily living—their ability to dress themselves, to bathe, to get to the bathroom, to eat. They had also been independent in somewhat more sophisticated functions such as driving, shopping, doing housework, paying bills, and all the other day-to-day activities necessary to keep going in contemporary society. But after one major illness, my father-in-law had stopped being robust and was now frail. He had dramatically deteriorated in almost all the fundamental activities of daily living: he was weak and could not walk well by himself outside the confines of his apartment; he needed help in dressing and showering. Not only had he become physically frail, but his memory had begun to fail him. Before his illness, this had been a minor problem for which he had been able to compensate. But during his illness and hospitalization the problem was aggravated by depression and no doubt at least transiently worsened as a result of general anesthesia, sleeping pills, and pain medication, and after he returned home his impaired memory and judgment became alarmingly evident. It was hard even for me, a physician with ample experience in the problems of the elderly, to accept: my father-in-law had not only become frail, he had also joined ranks with the multitude of octogenarians whose cognitive function was declining.

My mother-in-law was rapidly moving from being robust to being frail, although the full physical impact of her illness had not yet hit. Apart from a nagging pain in her back and abdomen, she felt reasonably well. She was still fully independent in her own care, though her long history of leaving the driving to her husband, coupled with intense anxiety surrounding driving, impaired her ability to get around. Her only clear and present problem was that she did not have the stamina to care for her husband unassisted. I anticipated, however, that she would soon need someone to take care of her. Her pain would probably get more severe as the tumor in her abdomen compressed other vital structures. She might develop nausea and vomiting along with her poor appetite as the metastases to her liver proliferated. She would lose weight; she would become weak. I knew with devastating certainty that in the relatively near future, she would pass from being robust to being frail and then would enter yet another stage where she would be among the dying.

As long as my in-laws had been vigorous, it seemed perfectly clear that the goals of their medical care should be the same as they had always been: to cure disease and to ameliorate suffering. Once they started on a downward slide, the goals of medical treatment began to change. Maintaining their independence and their dignity, keeping them in their own home, helping them with their walking, optimizing their ability to care for themselves and to continue to interact with friends and with us, their family, began to be more important than sheer survival. The effect of medical treatment on quality of life became ever more important. If chemotherapy existed for her cancer, how would it make my mother-in-law feel? How would it affect her ability to stay home with her husband? Would the possible benefits of treatment outweigh the burdens? I knew that when my father-in-law's cognitive function declined further and when my mother-in-law came closer to the end, the goal of medical care would change again. It would shift toward maximizing their comfort, away from treatment and toward palliation.

The goals I have just outlined were of course my goals. My husband's parents had not even begun to think about what would make sense for them as they entered the twilight of life. But I was more convinced than ever that my goals were actually their goals as well, and in fact would be almost everyone's goals if they understood what faced them as they traveled through old age. The reason that people often do not know how to think about how much and what kind of medical care to request is that they know little of the realities they will face until they are in the midst of a crisis. This book is an effort to help people imagine the kinds of situations they or their parents will be confronting as they enter their seventies, eighties, and nineties.

Patients in general and older patients in particular are increasingly being asked to make decisions about their health care. In accordance with the prevailing bioethical thinking, the patient's autonomy is paramount in deciding how much medical care and what kind of medical care are acceptable. Patients are expected to choose among alternative treatments on the basis of their personal preferences and values; they are expected to decide whether to forgo potentially beneficial treatments on the basis of their assessment of their own quality of life with and without the treatment; they are asked about whether they would wish to be resuscitated should their heart stop beating. Older patients, in whom these kinds of issues arise very commonly, are often unprepared to think about such issues. When they are acutely ill, they may be too frightened or in too much distress to think clearly. If their cognitive function is impaired, they may not be able to think about complex issues at all. I think it would be tremendously helpful to establish a framework in advance for thinking about the issues: not to have predetermined answers to all the questions that could conceivably arise, but to have sufficient understanding of what lies in store to be able to think about the questions when they do arise. By sufficient understanding I mean an awareness not only of the kinds of acute problems that may develop, but of what the treatment is likely to entail, given the underlying state of health of the patient. For contrary to much of the current discussion of limitation of treatment, curtailing treatment has a place not just in the event of terminal illness, not just when the patient's condition is deemed by him or her to be "worse than death," but also in many other circumstances. My father-in-law, for instance, regards his present condition as quite tolerable. But if he again developed problems for which surgery was recommended as the "best" option, he might well decline surgery if an alternative approach existed, even if that alternative was somewhat less likely to cure or alleviate his new problem. He had been so debilitated by his recent operation and took such a long time to recover that he was of the opinion that he might well prefer medical to surgical treatment in the future, even if it meant a lesser chance of surviving.

This kind of rehearsal of what might happen, this survey of possible trajectories as life winds down, would be unnecessarily painful if the probability of actually having to face decisions about medical care were small. Illness and disability in the elderly population are unfortunately extremely common, with little prospect for significant improvement in the near future. As people age, the fraction who can function independently gets smaller and smaller: only 9 percent of individuals in the community who are between ages 65 and 74 need help in one or more activities of daily living, but this rises to 14 percent for people 75 to 84 and soars to 31 percent for people

85 and over.[1] Dementia, a general term for progressive, usually irreversible cognitive decline, which includes Alzheimer's disease as well as a potpourri of other disorders, also increases dramatically in prevalence with age. While only 5 percent of those over 65 are demented, this rises to at least 20 percent in the population over 80, with some studies finding rates as high as 47 percent in community-dwelling elders over 85.[2] Hospitalization rates, another marker for the burden of disease, also rise with age. People over 65, who constitute 12 percent of the population, account for 30 percent of all hospital discharges; people over 75, who represent 5 percent of the population, constitute 16 percent of all hospital discharges.[3] And the death rate among individuals aged 65–74 is 2.6 percent, rising to 6.1 percent among those aged 75–84 and climbing to 15.0 percent in those 85 and over.[4]

The importance of having an approach to thinking about medical care for the elderly should be clear enough when we realize the prevalence both of acute illness and of underlying physical and intellectual impairment in older people. The urgency of having guidelines is even more apparent when we look at the rate of growth of the elderly population. The statistics are quoted often, yet they are so startling as to deserve repetition: 25.5 million Americans, or 11 percent of the population, were over 65 in 1980; 2.2 million, or 1 percent, were 85 or older. If we compare these percentages to those at the turn of the century, the growth is stunning: a mere 4 percent of the population were over 65 in 1900, and a barely measurable 0.2 percent over 85. If we then look into the future, we find the growth continuing at a remarkable rate: by 2020, the best estimates are that there will be 51.4 million people over 65, constituting 17 percent of the population, including 7.1 million people aged 85 or over (2.4 percent of the population).[5]

Coming up with a practical way of thinking about treating medical problems in the elderly is crucial because of the magnitude of the problem but also because of the enormity of the cost. The figures on health care expenditures are every bit as dramatic as the figures on population. Medical costs have been rising far faster than the inflation rate. Moreover, the elderly tend to be the sickest members of the population and therefore consume a disproportionate share of total health care resources. Statistics for the mid-1980s show that individuals over 65 accounted for $120 billion of the total health care costs, or one-third of health care expenditures.[6] While predictions of future costs are highly speculative, they are nonetheless useful approximations. Economists claim that Medicare spending for the elderly will double by 2020.[7]

If costs were high but outcomes were uniformly favorable, we as a society might be willing to accept even an extremely high price tag for the medical care of the elderly. But the data on the effectiveness of the health care provided to elderly people are far from clearcut. Much of the increase in life expectancy is attributable to public health measures and changes in living conditions unrelated to medicine.[8] To the extent that increased longevity is related to medical care, the primary contributors appear to be changes in diet and other life-style factors. The role of medical care in prolonging life in people who have reached old age is even less clear. We do know that while the quantity of life is greater than it used to be, the quality is often disappointing. Older people suffer from more chronic diseases and face greater limitations in their activities than ever before.[9] Those who survive into their late eighties are at high risk of developing dementia. And although there is no readily available means of measuring the dissatisfaction of the public with the procedure-oriented style of medical practice routinely used in virtually all patients, numerous testimonials in the media decry the "torture" to which elderly relatives have been subjected.[10] Popular support for living wills and other advance directives also derives in part from the perception that older individuals need to protect themselves from the excessively invasive tendencies of physicians.[11]

Not surprisingly, given the dimensions of the problem, public debate over how to provide medical care for the elderly is growing. But the major contributors to the debate are economists and philosophers. The economists focus on how to allocate care and how to achieve greater efficiency, addressing such questions as whether rationing medical care is necessary[12] and the relative merits of different kinds of health care delivery systems in terms of achieving cost savings.[13] Philosophers are concerned with similar themes— rationing, models of health care delivery—but evaluate them from the point of view of justice, or a discussion of what constitutes a good life, or a hierarchy of ethical principles.[14] Philosophers also address the micro as well as the macro or policy issues: the question of how individual physicians and patients should approach health care for the elderly. Biomedical ethicists agree that decisions about the kind or amount of medical care a patient should receive ought to be made by the individual patient, on the basis of his or her personal values. The patient's choice (or that of a surrogate if the patient cannot choose for himself) should be informed by technical information provided by his physician and made within the constraints set by national policy, but it is the patient's preferences that should be paramount in determining medical decisions.[15] My view as a physician is that in order to make personal choices or to formulate health care policy for the elderly, we need to start with a shared understanding of the reality of being old and sick. At least as important as religious beliefs or personal taste or abstract ideas about the sanctity of life is an intimate grasp of what it is like to be old and ill. Only by grappling with the experience of illness, by seeking to feel the texture of that experience, can individuals hope to make reasonable choices about what kind of care they would want for themselves or for others. And only if we start with a deep understanding of what being sick is like can we hope to reach a consensus on what kind of health policy is appropriate for the elderly.

There is no single reality of being old and sick: the elderly are a heterogeneous group, and old people can move rapidly from vigorous health to a state of weakness and dependence in an alarmingly short period of time, as happened to my mother-in-law. I find it useful to think of older people in terms of their capacities, their ability to function independently. At one extreme are the robust, healthy elderly, people who have no limitations on their activities of daily life even though they may have a number of chronic medical illnesses and might take a variety of pills to keep going. At the other extreme are those elderly people who are dying. It is becoming harder to define who is dying, in large measure because of our growing technological capacities, but there are still a number of people who are clearly near death regardless of what medical interventions they submit to. In between the robust and the dying are the frail elderly, those whose medical problems are typically multiple and debilitating, individuals who need help with such basics as getting dressed or bathing. A final group, which I feel deserves special attention both because it is rapidly growing in size and because of its unique character, consists of people with dementia. These older people cannot function independently because of mental rather than physical incapacity.

My journey into the world of sickness in the elderly begins with those who suffer from the great geriatric plague, dementia. The old person who has lost much of his capacity to think and reason is a fitting starting point not because dementia is universal among the elderly—it certainly is not—but because the plight of the demented person who develops an acute medical problem so poignantly illustrates why we need a context in which to place decisions about medical care for the elderly. The situation of the demented person who becomes physically ill highlights the need to look at the interaction between the acute illness, the treatment of the acute illness, and the underlying status of the patient, before formulating a reasonable course of action. The patients I describe come from different circumstances: one is a nursing home patient with no family; one lives in a nursing home and has an extremely involved family; one lives at home with an elaborate caretaking system. Each of them raises questions about the kind of care that is most appropriate. Are painful or invasive techniques too burdensome to be justified in demented patients? Is conventional medical care as effective in this group as in other patients, or does it carry with it a series of perhaps unacceptable risks? Are families in the best position to speak on behalf of relatives who have lost the capacity to reason and to make their preferences known? How helpful are advance directives in this setting?

From the disturbing and for many alien world of the demented patient, I will move to the more familiar world of the robust elderly. Just because we all know vigorous older individuals does not mean that we have a good intuitive grasp of the issues they face when they get sick. I will tell the stories of several independent, mentally intact older people who developed serious illnesses and focus on the dilemmas with which they struggled. Does aggressive medical care make sense for this group? Is there any age beyond which techno-logical interventions are not warranted? Can patients always be expected to know in advance what kind of treatment they prefer? Are there certain kinds of treatments that are uniformly poorly tol-erated by older people, for either technical or emotional reasons?

From the robust elderly, I will travel next to the realm of the dying. This is the group on which most of the discussion about limiting treatment focuses. But is it always clear who is dying? At what point does it make sense for the goal of care to become pal-liation? What kind of institutional environment is most conducive to an exclusive focus on comfort rather than cure? Is there a role for assisted suicide or euthanasia in dying patients?

Finally, I will talk about patients who are neither robust nor dying nor demented, the group commonly referred to as the frail elderly. I will tell the stories of people whose plight is seldom publicly dis-cussed: a woman who regards her life as worse than death even though she is not terminally ill; a woman who discovers that nursing home care makes her life eminently worth living; and a man who learns the hard way that hospital care is fraught with risk.

On the basis of this tour of the old and sick, I will suggest broad guidelines for what constitutes a sensible approach to medical care for each group. Within this overarching framework there is ample room for flexibility, for patients together with their families and their physicians to come up with individualized decisions about care. But the decisions will constitute variations on a theme rather than radically different styles of treatment. For these suggested guidelines to be implemented, both conceptual change in the way doctors and patients think about medical care and institutional change in the way doctors practice medicine will be essential. I will close with a brief foray into the world we will need to create if the proposed approach is to be implemented—a world with new kinds of nursing homes, more inpatient hospice facilities, fewer hospitals, and new infirmaries, a world in which quality as well as quantity of life figures into cost-benefit calculations and where physicians as well as patients are comfortable with sophisticated but low-technology medical care.

It is my hope that these stories of illness, with their many permutations of fact, of family, and of fortune, will help patients, potential patients, and relatives of patients to imagine what treatment would be like in their particular situation. My book is too late to help my in-laws: my mother-in-law died of her overwhelming cancer before I had even completed the first draft. But I hope that once others can conceive of what the future holds, their choice about which path to tread will become, if not self-evident, at least reasonably straightforward. If more and more of us come to hold a common view of what aging and experiencing illness are all about, we as a society may move toward a consensus about the kind of medical care that makes sense for elderly people in various circumstances. Despite our differences in religion, socioeconomic class, education, or occupation, we may discover that we have more in common than we thought.

❖ 1 ❖

Robbed of Mind and Memory:
The Demented Elderly

By the time my son was two, he knew that a visit to the pediatrician's office meant trouble. I remember when he stood clutching my hand in the foyer leading to his doctor's office, feverish and miserable, and gallantly offered that I go ahead and see the doctor myself—he would wait for me. He knew that if he went in, he would be prodded and poked; at worst he would be given an injection, at best a foul-tasting medicine to take for the next ten days, eternity to a two-year-old. Yet of course I insisted that he go in, knowing full well that he would gag on his doctor's tongue depressor and recoil from the cold stethoscope and cry when his ears were examined. The price was small for what I knew would be a definitive diagnosis and cure.

The power of medicine to heal is so intimately entwined with its capacity to cause discomfort that we are often suspicious of medical treatment that is not at all noxious. We tolerate the bitter pill that physicians prescribe because we know it is in our best interest to swallow it. We subject our children to examinations and medical interventions because we recognize that even severe pain is a worthwhile price to pay for their future health and well-being. But is there ever a point at which vigorous medical treatment no longer makes sense—not because it is incapable of producing the desired biological effect, not because it is too expensive, but rather because it is simply too much for the patient to bear? In particular, are there times when people should reject medical treatment that is extremely invasive because they are in the final stage of their lives—not necessarily dying, but close enough to the end to feel that burdensome treatment may no longer be for them?

The dilemma of when to stop treating, or when to provide less than maximally intensive care, is never more poignant than with the elderly person who has Alzheimer's disease or one of several other types of that devastating, chronic, progressive disorder known as dementia. Dementia, the gradual loss of multiple facets of the mind such as memory, language, and judgment, robs people of their ability to understand what is happening to them when they get sick. Illness becomes as incomprehensible to these patients as its treatment. Moreover, the future they are vouchsafed if they are successfully cured of pneumonia or appendicitis is one of relentless decline. If they live long enough, they will likely pass from a state of mild forgetfulness to apathy and incontinence, and ultimately to a bedbound existence. I was just beginning my career as a physician when I was forced to deal with the perils of trying to give what is typically regarded as good medical care to a severely demented patient.

When Treatment Turns to Torment

It was late at night when I was called to the emergency room to see a patient who was being admitted to the hospital. I was the intern who would provide the majority of the hands-on care while he was in the hospital. I was told that the patient was 85 years old and had a fever and "altered mental status." This last meant he was confused, perhaps agitated, perhaps belligerent.

In the far corner of the emergency room, behind a partly drawn curtain, my patient lay on a stretcher. He was curled up in a fetal position, his legs drawn up to his chest. His right arm was restrained to prevent him from pulling out the intravenous needle which had been inserted after multiple attempts into a narrow, tortuous vein in his left arm. His eyes were half closed. I looked briefly at the emergency room chart: a nursing home resident, no family, Alzheimer's disease. Unable to feed or dress himself, incontinent, unable to carry on a conversation, even when at his best. Noted that day to be sleepier than usual, pushed away the spoon when being fed. Found to have a fever of 103. No cough, no diarrhea, no complaints of pain. Previously in good physical health. Receives pills to control his agitation, but no other medications.

I approached him. "Mr. Brown?" I said. There was no response. I double-checked the emergency room sheet: the name was indeed Brown. I looked at his wrist identification bracelet. It was the right patient. I tried again, louder, in deference to the fact that many elderly people are hard of hearing. He moaned slightly. I rubbed him on the chest, in an attempt to arouse him from stupor. He lifted the arm that was not tied down and tried to brush me away, as if I were an insect buzzing around him. "Mr. Brown," I said, "open your eyes." Even people whose capacity to understand spoken language is markedly diminished as a result of neurological disease can usually follow this kind of simple command. He opened his eyes briefly and then closed them again. This time I tried verbal and physical stimulation simultaneously: I rubbed on his chest and asked loudly that he open his eyes. He opened his eyes and mumbled "go away." I made one final attempt. I introduced myself as his doctor. I told him my name. I told him he had a fever and the nurses at the nursing home were concerned about him. He dozed off.

Clearly I would not be able to elicit a history from this patient. I proceeded with the physical examination. I discovered that he remembered some four-letter words when I tried taking his blood pressure and a stream of profanity issued from his half-open mouth. The physical examination was only marginally more successful than the history. I attempted to look at his eyes with my ophthalmoscope in search of an abnormality that would indicate he had a brain tumor or hemorrhage to account for his lethargy. He had dense cataracts in both eyes that literally clouded the view. He refused to open his mouth to permit me to look for evidence of infection there—a dental abscess, a throat inflammation. I got a quick peek inside when he yawned, enough to determine only that he was toothless. An adequate lung exam was equally impossible. For that he needed to sit up and take deep breaths while I listened with my stethoscope. And so it went on down to his toes: I could not properly feel his abdomen because of the contractures in his legs—he was bent at the hips, his legs could not be straightened out. I could at least visually inspect his skin, looking for rashes or sores. He had none.

The physical examination, such as it was, did not provide an explanation for his fever. Perhaps the laboratory data would yield the answer. Surely those tests were objective, quantifiable, definitive. Mr. Brown had had a single view taken in the emergency room with a portable machine rather than with the superior technique available in the X-ray suite. He had not taken a deep breath while the X-ray was taken, so his lungs were compressed rather than fully expanded, making interpretation difficult. The radiologist could tell me there was a possibility of pneumonia at the bottom of the right lung. But it might be scar tissue, residual damage from prior lung disease. It might be fluid, which could be due to an infection, cancer, or heart failure. And it was equally possible that it might be an artifact that would disappear if Mr. Brown could cooperate for a better-quality X-ray.

The emergency room physician had obtained a urine test by inserting a catheter through Mr. Brown's penis into his bladder, since Mr. Brown was unable to provide a specimen on demand. His urine was loaded with white blood cells and bacteria, but elderly men often have bacteria in their urine at all times. Their presence did not implicate the urinary tract as the source of the fever.

With no certain explanation for the fever at hand, I proceeded to do more tests: first, blood cultures, looking for bacteria in the blood itself. Blood cultures are in principle not very difficult to obtain. All I had to do was to wash Mr. Brown's arm with a disinfectant solution, draw blood, and then do the same thing again fifteen minutes later. But Richard Brown's veins tended to collapse—they seemed to recede from view when approached with a needle. His skin was thick, so the needle hurt going in. A nurse held him down as I tried, several times, to draw his blood. He was awake now, and yelling: "Don't touch me . . . Cut that out." Forty-five minutes later, I was able to send the requisite two sets of blood cultures to the laboratory.

The culture results would not be available for a day or two. In the meantime, there was one more test left to do, a lumbar puncture, to determine if Mr. Brown had meningitis, a severe but rare infection of the lining surrounding the brain and spinal cord.

I wheeled Mr. Brown up to his room before doing the lumbar puncture and enlisted the help of a nurse and another doctor. We turned our patient on his side, holding his legs firmly and tying down both his arms. The nurse spoke soothingly to him. "It's all right, Richard. It's almost over." It wasn't almost over. Mr. Brown's spine was curved, making it difficult to locate the perfect spot into which to insert the needle. Just when I thought I might have found the right spot, he moved. "No! Don't do that!" he screamed. I told him it was just a test to find out what was wrong with him, that it wouldn't really hurt because I had given him a local anesthetic. I was talking to myself—the words were meaningless to him. Again and again I inserted the needle, waiting for a few drops of cerebrospinal fluid to drip out, signifying that the needle had entered the sheath just outside the nerves of the spinal column that contained the protective fluid. "Ow!" he yelped as I tried a new spot. I screened out the yells and concentrated on the bony prominences of his back with the tough skin between them. On the fourth try, I succeeded. The fluid was clear. There were no bacteria or white blood cells in it when I examined it under the microscope—nothing to suggest meningitis.

I started Mr. Brown on intravenous antibiotics for a probable urinary tract infection. Within a day his temperature was down to normal. In another day he was alert and no longer excessively sleepy. He started eating again. The blood cultures were negative. After three days I switched him to oral antibiotics. The following day I discharged him back to his nursing home. Nobody had visited him while he was in the hospital.

I took care of many patients like Mr. Brown as an intern at an inner-city hospital. Not one of them proved to have meningitis. A few did have a bloodstream infection, but in most cases they were already being treated with the appropriate antibiotic. Some of the patients died, despite use of the optimal antibiotics. All of them found the tests and therapies to which they were subjected incomprehensible. They were frightened and uncomfortable. For Mr. Brown and the many others like him who enter the hospital, whose dementia is irreversible and who in their eighties are near the end of their lives, I was not at all convinced that the benefit of conventional treatment warranted the anguish I was inflicting on them. I had the nagging feeling I was tormenting them.

If the plight of Richard Brown were a rare phenomenon, I would regard the entire episode as painful and tragic, but unavoidable. Unfortunately, dementia is far from rare. An estimated 5 percent of individuals over 65 who live at home have severe dementia, and as many as 10 percent have mild dementia.[1] In the population over age 85 who live at home, most estimates indicate that roughly 20 percent are demented,[2] though recent studies suggest that the frequency may be even higher, perhaps as high as 47 percent.[3] At least 50 percent of nursing home patients have dementia.[4] Using conservative estimates, this yields a grand total of 1.3 million people with severe dementia and another 2.8 million people with mild to moderate dementia. By contrast, the clinical situation in which limiting medical care is most hotly debated is persistent vegetative state, a form of coma, which currently afflicts a mere 10,000 individuals in the United States. Deaths from cancer, the other condition in which withholding treatment is often considered, total 475,000 per year.

What I would have preferred to do for Richard Brown would have been to treat what was statistically the most likely cause of his fever, his urinary tract infection, without subjecting him to the indignity of further testing that served only to exclude, or rule out, more obscure possible etiologies. I would have given him antibiotics, by mouth if he were alert enough to swallow, by injection if not, preferably back at the nursing home. In short, I favored taking the small but not negligible risk of treating him with the wrong antibiotic or for the wrong disease. Given the cost to Mr. Brown of gaining that additional bit of certainty, in light of his poor long-term prognosis whether he survived his bout of infection or not, it was a chance I thought reasonable to take. But was the physician the one to make such a decision?[5]

The prevailing contemporary view is that it is the patient who should make decisions about limiting care. Patient autonomy, or the right of patients to decide for themselves, is the centerpiece of contemporary medical ethics.[6] Demented patients, however, are by definition unable to participate in any but the most simplistic discussions about their medical care because of their intellectual limitations. A widely touted solution to this dilemma is the use of advance directives.

Advance directives, quite simply, are documents that permit individuals while of sound mind to specify what kinds of medical care they would want in a variety of circumstances. They may take one of several forms: they may be living wills (usually general statements declining heroic measures at the end of life); they may designate a proxy, or surrogate decision maker, who is empowered to make decisions on the patient's behalf; or they may attempt to list in detail, for each of several well-defined clinical conditions, exactly what interventions an individual would want.

The problem with living wills is that they almost always apply to imminently terminal illness, not to chronic diseases such as Alzheimer's disease. One standard form for creating a living will, for instance, specifies that it will take effect in the event that "I should have an injury, disease, or illness, which is certified in writing to be a terminal condition by two physicians who have personally examined me; and in the opinion of those physicians the application of life-sustaining procedures would serve only to unnaturally postpone or prolong the moment of my death and to unnaturally postpone or prolong the dying process."[7] A simpler form, but with basically the same message, reads in part: "If . . . the situation should arise in which there is no reasonable expectation of my recovery from extreme physical or mental disability, I direct that I be allowed to die and not be kept alive by medication, artificial means or 'heroic' measures."[8] An irreversible mental disability might include dementia, although it more likely was meant to refer to persistent vegetative states. Even if it is taken to include dementia, what it addresses are life-saving measures, not routine care for new medical problems such as the treatment of infection in Richard Brown. This is quite clear from the suggested additional provision: "Measures of artificial life support in the face of impending death that are especially abhorrent to me are: (a) electrical or mechanical resuscitation of my heart when it has stopped beating; (b) nasogastric tube feedings when I am paralyzed and no longer able to swallow; (c) mechanical respiration by machine when my brain can no longer sustain my own breathing." There is no doubt that this will is meant to guide physicians at the time of impending death.

Even far more explicit and extensive advance directives deal only with patients who are terminally ill, where death is expected in weeks or at most months, or who are irreversibly comatose.[9] They do not touch on what kind of medical care individuals would want for themselves should they develop an irreversible dementia that will lead to death only after a period of years.

Not only do few advance directives explicitly mention dementia (presumably a remediable defect of such instruments), but few mentally intact people actually consider what it would be like to have Alzheimer's disease. Aside from a vague sense of dread, they have thought neither about what medical treatment would be like for them if they were demented, nor about what kinds of limitations they would wish. Perhaps this will change as dementia becomes a less taboo subject. At present, physicians seldom tell patients with Alzheimer's disease their diagnosis; or they may employ euphemisms such as "cognitive impairment" or "memory problem." The prevailing situation is not unlike that of cancer in the 1950s and early 1960s, at which time a landmark study revealed that 90 percent of clinicians did not disclose the diagnosis of cancer to their patients.[10] When the study was repeated in the late 1970s, 97 percent of physicians told their patients they had cancer.[11] Thus dementia in general and Alzheimer's disease in particular are what cancer was thirty or forty years ago—the great unmentionable, though there is some movement in the direction of greater disclosure of the diagnosis.[12] In no small measure because of the greater openness in discussing cancer, individuals can now imagine what it would be like to have untreatable, often painful, metastatic cancer and to plan for that eventuality. However, they know little about dementia, are faced with powerful psychological barriers to thinking about "losing their minds," and, not surprisingly, can offer little guidance to their physicians about what approach to medical care would make sense should they develop this dreaded and mysterious ailment.

The final problem with advance directives is that despite the publicity they have received, relatively few patients fill them out. In a survey conducted by the American Medical Association, 15 percent of people were found to have a living will.[13] Only 25 percent of Americans draw up ordinary wills, so the chance that greater numbers will complete a medical advance directive is slim.[14]

If patients with dementia are incapable of stating their preferences and only rarely leave explicit directives applicable to the case of dementia, to what other sources can physicians turn? The obvious answer is that family members of demented patients have ideas on how their relatives should be treated. Family members can be trusted to have ideas, but whether their ideas reflect what demented individuals would have wanted for themselves, or even what is in the best interest of demented patients, is another matter.

The Limits of Family Decision Making

Tony Londino had always been close to his mother. He told me a bit about their relationship at the time of her first checkup in my office, when she was 76. Tony's father had died young, leaving Maria Londino to raise Tony and his two sisters by herself. His mother had worked in a garment factory to support the family. When that job proved too inflexible, not allowing her to be home with her children after school, she took a variety of odd jobs. Then Tony's older sister became ill, and his mother stopped working in order to care for her. He never knew what was wrong with his sister, but he dropped out of school so he could get a job. His sister died and his mother was devastated. Tony continued working, providing at age 16 both financial and emotional support for his mother. He went to night school to get a high school diploma, and managed to procure a clerical job at a large export firm. Tony's younger sister married and moved back to Italy, but Tony remained a bachelor and lived with his mother. Over the years he remained with the same company and gradually rose a few notches in the hierarchy.

The Londinos lived in a small two-bedroom apartment in a working-class suburb. Every five years they went on vacation to Italy together to see family. In the evenings they played cards; on Sundays they went to church. Mrs. Londino kept house for her son. They lived a simple life and, in Tony's words, were devoted to each other.

When Maria Londino turned 75, she began to be noticeably forgetful. Tony did not think much of her memory loss, attributing it to old age. But when he turned 60 and she turned 78, he took early retirement to be able to care for her. I was surprised because sons only rarely play such an active caretaking role. Most of the personal help provided by families is performed by women: wives, daughters, and daughters-in-law, in that order.[15] Tony explained that he had recruited a personal attendant from his church, but she continually insisted that Maria belonged in a nursing home. Unable to find help who were up to the task, Tony decided to take over himself. For two years he cooked, cleaned, shopped, and took his mother on excursions. Whenever he brought her for appointments, she was clean and neat. I suggested they might both benefit from sending her to an adult day care program: she would socialize with other people her age and he would have a break for a few hours each day. Tony came up with an extensive list of excuses for why he could not possibly let her go to day care. But when she became incontinent, Tony grudgingly put her in a nursing home. He could not bring himself to change her soiled underclothes or to bathe her. He told me he sometimes wished he were a woman so he would be able to give his mother personal care without humiliating her. He just did not feel he could give her the care she deserved.

Maria adjusted to life in the nursing home quite easily. At first she seemed to brighten up and smile when Tony came to visit. She always appeared to be glad of his company but ceased distinguishing him from other friendly figures in her life. I was not convinced she knew who he was. She did not remember his name. Sometimes she called him her nurse, which was not too far off; sometimes she referred to him as her cabdriver or teacher. I was uncertain whether her errors reflected the word-finding difficulty characteristic of Alzheimer's disease or whether she simply did not know who he was. My suspicion was that it was both.

Tony had much more difficulty adjusting to the nursing home. He visited daily and was never satisfied with his mother's care. He wanted her to be put to bed when she was up and to be up when she was in bed. He was angry that her legs were swollen and could not accept that they would remain swollen unless she wore support stockings—she wouldn't—and unless she kept them elevated—she didn't. He wanted her to attend bingo even though she could no longer follow the game and disrupted it by pacing and by taking the other residents' cards and chits.

Immediately after Maria's admission to the nursing home, I attempted to discuss the issue of cardiopulmonary resuscitation with Tony. I had once before tried to talk about what kind of medical care she should receive if she became very ill, but Tony had not wanted to discuss theoretical problems. He was a practical man. Since federal legislation, the Patient Self-Determination Act, requires that all patients admitted to a nursing home be asked if they have or are interested in having a living will or health care proxy,[16] the move to the nursing home was a convenient opportunity to raise the issue again. Maria Londino neither had a living will nor had she designated a formal health care proxy, but Tony was her unofficial surrogate. I portrayed for him the grim odds of successful resuscitation in the event of a cardiac arrest in the nursing home.[17] Despite the statistics, Tony insisted that if his mother's heart stopped beating and she stopped breathing, everything should be tried. "God will take her when He's ready," Tony told me. I told him that even the Pope had affirmed that extraordinary measures were not morally necessary in the eyes of the Church,[18] but Tony was not persuaded. I asked him if his mother had ever discussed her wishes. He answered that she had been a deeply religious woman who never wanted to be a burden to anyone, and who believed that when her time came, she should go quietly. I suggested that ventilators, defibrillators, and the other equipment used during a cardiac arrest were decidedly human interventions and that allowing nature to take its course meant sparing his mother technological intervention. Tony did not see it that way. I entered a note in the medical record indicating that if Maria Londino had a cardiac arrest, resuscitation should be attempted.

Maria remained in good physical health for the next two years. Her dementia, however, relentlessly progressed. Her speech became garbled. She became restless and paced the halls ceaselessly. She became paranoid. Ultimately, her balance began to fail in tandem with her judgment and she fell repeatedly. When she could no longer walk independently with safety, she spent much of the day in a reclining chair.

The cruelest development for Tony was to see his mother unable to feed herself. The complicated sequence of chewing, pushing food to the back of the mouth, and swallowing was too much for her. She pocketed the food, storing it in her cheeks like a chipmunk. She spat the food out. Her nutritional status declined, despite special supplemental milkshakes. I asked Tony whether he wanted us to surgically insert a gastrostomy tube (G-tube) into his mother's stomach in order to feed her.

Maria's primary nurse, who saw her daily, was vehemently opposed to a G-tube. She told Tony that she thought Maria was frightened by her inability to understand what was happening in her environment and her inability to communicate her needs. The nurse was convinced that Maria's difficult behavior—her spitting, banging her shoe, and episodic screaming—was a reflection of her intense frustration with herself and her surroundings. She reminded Tony that when Maria had briefly had a catheter in her bladder she had pulled it out herself, which the nurse took as a sign that she did not want anything medical done to her. I was not convinced. Fully two-thirds of all people with Alzheimer's disease manifest disturbed and disturbing behavior. I was similarly reluctant to place much weight on the fact that Maria had pulled out tubes before. I suspected that all she was trying to tell us was that she did not like hoses dangling from her nose or worming their way into her private parts. In the absence of any comprehension of what the tube is or why it is there, I do not think anyone could seriously regard the patient's tugging on the tube as an informed decision to forgo treatment. I did agree that Maria showed no evidence of deriving either pleasure or meaning from life. Some people with Alzheimer's disease cannot remember much and cannot do much for themselves, but they smile and are docile. Maria did not smile and she was not docile. She kicked and scratched her way through each monotonous day.

Tony told me that he could not let his mother starve to death. I assured him that she would not suffer if she only ate and drank whatever small amount she wished. She would not, after all, be deprived of food. She would be offered plenty, and the nursing assistants understood they needed to allow ample time to feed Maria. The staff would give her snacks, and Tony was encouraged to bring in any special treats she might enjoy. There was no reason to believe that Maria would experience hunger if she failed to consume the recommended daily allowance of each of the major food groups. In fact, she would more than likely gradually become dehydrated, and as the salt and waste products in her blood rose as a result of dehydration, she would slip into a stupor and then coma. Dehydration, I told Tony, was a natural anesthetic. Eventually, if Maria truly stopped eating and drinking, she would fade away. It was not a bad way to go, I commented, and end-stage Alzheimer's disease was a lethal illness.

Tony acknowledged that perhaps his mother would not suffer without a gastrostomy tube, but he was not going to be the one to sentence her to death. I tried to tell him that it was her disease that would cause her death, not Tony's decision about a feeding tube, but he refused to discuss the situation further. Reluctantly, I admitted Maria to the hospital where, under anesthesia, a surgeon made an incision into her abdomen and passed an endoscope through her mouth into her stomach, permitting him to visualize the placement of a rubber tube directly into the stomach. She returned to the nursing home the next day.

Once Maria had a G-tube in place, she began gaining weight. The nursing assistants were delighted that they no longer had to spend so much time feeding her; instead, the nurse hooked the feeding tube up to a bottle of a special formula and let it drip in, much like an intravenous solution. Tony associated feeding with nurturing, but this kind of feeding was its antithesis.

Despite her improved nutritional status, Maria developed pneumonia. She became feverish, short of breath, and lethargic. I called Tony and told him we had several options. We could send her to the hospital where she would receive intravenous antibiotics. We could keep her at the nursing home and give her antibiotics through her G-tube or via injection. Or we could keep her at the nursing home and make her comfortable using oxygen and Tylenol, a far from unprecedented practice in nursing homes.[19]

Tony did not hesitate for a moment. He said he wanted her rushed to the nearest hospital. I attempted to suggest that pneumonia was often successfully treated in the nursing home setting, and that if his mother were transferred she would become even more agitated than usual. He was not interested. Maria went to the hospital where she was restrained, sedated, and acquired a deep bed sore on her buttocks.

Over the next few months, Tony became more demanding—in the view of the staff, more unreasonable than ever. He insisted that a physical therapist work with her on exercises, though her memory and comprehension were far too impaired for her to retain anything she was shown, and her legs were too contracted for her to benefit from exercise. He demanded that I draw her blood to check for anemia because she looked pale to him. He hung around the nurses' station, clamoring for her diaper to be changed or asking endless questions: what was her weight, how was her blood pressure, should a surgeon look at her bed sore.

On her eighty-third birthday, Maria's nurse noticed that her lungs were congested. She was breathing rapidly and her pulse was thready. I came in to see her and found that she was in pulmonary edema: her lungs were filled with fluid as a result of a failing heart. Her electrocardiogram confirmed that she was having a massive heart attack. I reached Tony at home and told him that his mother's condition was precarious. I was not optimistic that hospitalization could salvage her, but I did not even bother to suggest that we could treat her at the nursing home. I knew that if Maria died at the home, Tony would never forgive himself for failing to insist that she have the ostensible benefit of hospital care.

Twelve hours later, Maria Londino died. She died in the coronary care unit, tied down, with a catheter in the artery of her wrist and another catheter threaded through her heart into the far reaches of her pulmonary circulation. She had had all the best that modern medicine had to offer, including a temporary pacemaker that was inserted when her heart rate had slowed to twenty beats a minute. The pacemaker kept on firing, but Maria's heart no longer responded.

Everyone involved in Maria Londino's care—the caretakers when she was at home, the nurses and aides at the nursing home, and myself—believed that her son Tony was truly dedicated to his mother. We also believed that the decisions he had made on her behalf about her medical care reflected his needs rather than her wishes and that those decisions were contrary to his mother's best interests. The nurses were variously hostile, angry, or frustrated in their dealings with Tony. They came to regard themselves as Maria's advocates, as her only chance of living out her life with a modicum of grace in a world gone amok trying to honor patient or family autonomy.

The nurses were convinced that Tony was not following his mother's express wishes because Tony had so much as admitted this was so. He confessed he had never talked with her much about what she would want if she were very ill, and he certainly had never broached the subject of medical care in the event of dementia. When pressed, Tony did recall that his mother had had a friend who developed Alzheimer's disease—or Old Timers' disease, as she called it—and that Maria had stopped visiting her friend because she found it too painful. Maria had, however, stated very clearly that she did not want to be a burden to anyone in her old age. She never defined precisely what she meant by being a burden, but she almost certainly meant that she did not want to be dependent on others for care. When Maria Londino's husband died, she vowed never to go on welfare and insisted on supporting her children herself, even when it meant holding down three different part-time jobs. Tony also reported that although his mother always wanted to feel in control of certain aspects of her life, such as her work and her family, she was quite fatalistic about sickness and death. Perhaps the only way she had made sense of her daughter's premature death was to believe that it was ordained by God. On those rare occasions when she talked about her own death—on her seventy-fifth birthday, when she announced that she had become an old woman and God would take her soon—she was peacefully resigned.

Tony, like many family members who are called upon to serve as surrogate decision makers, had a difficult time making medical decisions using substituted judgment, judgment based on what his mother would have wanted had she been able to speak for herself. A survey of the preferences of surrogate decision makers for severely demented nursing home patients found that in 70 percent of cases, the decisions were made independent of any previously expressed wishes of the patient.[20] Even if he had tried to decide about the G-tube or hospitalization for pneumonia by assessing what he thought his mother would want, he might well have guessed wrong. Comparisons between what patients say they want for themselves and what their spouses think they want[21] and between patients and their self-selected surrogates[22] have shown poor concordance.

Just because Tony Londino did not try to make decisions based on substituted judgment, and perhaps could not have used such a standard, does not mean that his views were contrary to his mother's best interests. There is, after all, currently no gold standard for determining just what Maria Londino's best interests were. The nurses believed that transferring Mrs. Londino to an acute care hospital for treatment of pneumonia would produce needless suffering. They regarded hospitalization in the setting of her imminent demise from a heart attack as inhumane. No majority view prevails on how aggressively to treat uncomprehending, elderly, demented patients because most people have not considered the question. There is some evidence that families of severely demented patients, when given a choice of alternative levels of care for their relatives, tend to select the least aggressive options. In one special care unit for dementia patients modeled on a hospice, families were offered a series of possible approaches to medical care: aggressive workup and treatment of acute conditions, including hospitalization and cardiopulmonary resuscitation (CPR); all of the above but without CPR; nursing home treatment of acute conditions with no CPR or transfer to the hospital; palliative care; or palliative care plus no artificial feeding. When given these choices, fully 63 percent favored palliation alone and another 35 percent favored nursing home treatment alone. Only one out of forty family members wanted hospital-level care in the event of acute illness.[23] On the other hand, another survey of families of severely demented nursing home patients found that they favored hospitalization of their family members in 63 percent of cases, admission to an intensive care unit in 75 percent of cases, and tube feeding in 36 percent of cases when such a course was recommended by a physician.[24] Thus there is no consensus on what constitutes the best interest of demented patients, though there is a trend toward limiting care. And at least in some settings, when the possible alternatives are spelled out in detail, family members of demented patients come to regard comfort measures as most consistent with best interests. In one poll, 91 percent of gerontologists (specialists in the elderly, including both physicians and non-physicians) and 90 percent of family members of demented patients regarded hospice-style care as appropriate for end-stage dementia.[25]

Tony Londino may have made poor decisions for his mother, but who could have made better decisions? Maria Londino might not have wanted a G-tube, had she imagined herself in a position of being too demented to eat, but does that imply that she would have wanted her nurses, or me, or anyone else to speak for her? Conceivably, many potential patients are willing to designate a surrogate simply because they would prefer to have someone they love attempt to judge their best interests rather than a stranger. They understand full well that those surrogates will not necessarily act as they would have, but nonetheless trust their judgment.

Unfortunately, although patients often wish to have surrogates make decisions for them, the prospective surrogates are sometimes ill-equipped for this new responsibility. Family members often face a conflict of interest: if they make medical care decisions for an incompetent relative that prolong that person's life, they will be faced with an emotional and sometimes a financial burden. On the other hand, if they vote against life-prolonging interventions, they may bear the burden of guilt for the rest of their lives.[26] The solution to this dilemma is to involve surrogates in certain kinds of medical decision making but as a society to reach a consensus about a reasonable approach to the care of the demented patient. Once society as a whole has established broad guidelines for care, such as deciding whether demented patients should be eligible for perpetual dialysis or chronic feeding tubes, then the kinds of decisions left for surrogates will be the narrower choices that truly are a matter of personal preference.

If some patients such as Richard Brown leave no clue as to what kind of care they wish to receive and have no family or friends to speak for them, and some patients such as Maria Londino have as surrogate decision makers family members whose choices reflect their personal interests rather than the best interests of the patient, how are we ever to come to a consensus? In part, the answer is a technical one: physicians need to define a standard of medical care for demented patients that represents something other than abandonment but that is different from the now conventional, maximally invasive approach to care.

The belief in the efficacy of modern medical care is so profound that we often fail to recognize that less technologically intensive approaches to treatment have a significant likelihood of succeeding. The essence of professional training is to learn what the single best treatment is and then to provide it. Studies of medical treatment typically attempt to elucidate which of various regimens is the best and then seek to supplant old remedies with new ones. Quality assurance strategies, which aim to define precisely what constitutes optimal care—which tests, which medications, what doses—also promote the view that there is a single right way to practice medicine by explicitly criticizing physicians for failing to adhere to a set protocol.[27]

The problem with routinely recommending a single, maximalist course of treatment is that this approach seriously overestimates the benefits of conventional care and underestimates the benefits of less aggressive care, particularly for frail, elderly patients. Standard treatment is often far less than uniformly successful. Among patients aged 75 or over admitted to an intensive care unit, fully 38 percent will die, despite maximal medical therapy, compared to considerably lower rates in younger age groups.[28] Contrary to commonsense expectations, a study of severely demented nursing home patients found no difference in survival rate between those patients who developed fever and were given antibiotics and those who developed fever and were treated with Tylenol.[29]

Not only is standard treatment less than perfectly effective, it is also associated with a significant risk of side effects, a risk that patients near the end of life may not be willing to take. In one hospital, 41 percent of patients over 70 experienced adverse consequences of hospitalization, compared to 9 percent of patients under 70.[30]

Conversely, physicians often fail to realize that the efficacy of treatments other than maximalist care is considerably greater than zero. For example, treatment of patients with chronic renal failure using diuretics and a low-protein diet rather than dialysis may be associated with a reasonably good quality of life. Selected patients with strokes[31] and heart attacks[32] have been successfully treated at home instead of in the hospital. And in the example of the nursing home patients with fever, not only is there a failure rate with antibiotics, there is a success rate with Tylenol.

In a few situations, physicians routinely offer alternative treatments that have roughly equivalent efficacy rates. Breast cancer is a case in which physicians are legally mandated to discuss the availability of mastectomy or lumpectomy plus radiation therapy.[33]

These options have similar but not identical cure rates, and the choice depends largely on how strongly the woman feels about breast preservation. In general, however, the choice physicians give patients or their surrogates is either to accept or to refuse treatment. When phrased this way, as a take-it-or-leave-it proposition, the choice offered adheres to the letter but not the spirit of patient involvement in decision making. Only in the relatively rare circumstances where life is perceived as truly worse than death will surrogates refuse treatment if they are offered a choice between doing something—and possibly permitting the patient to live—and doing nothing—and certainly causing the patient to die. "Doing nothing" carries with it the connotation of callous disregard. It sounds like abandonment. In fact, the alternative to maximalist intervention is almost never closing the door and leaving the patient to die.[34]

The Option of Intermediate-Level Care

Most families, when offered the possibility of intermediate-level care, will leap at the opportunity. A role for just this kind of approach came up shortly after Nadine Chang enrolled in my practice as a house call patient.

Nadine Chang was a 71-year-old woman who had formerly established and run her own business. She had been very successful and well respected in the Chinese-American community. Over a period of several years, she became increasingly forgetful and confused, conducting herself in an inappropriate manner. Previously very polite and courteous, she suddenly was rude to her clients and insulting to her employees. She became very demanding, insisting that the cashier in her store bring her tea and asking the clerk to drive her home. She began to dress in a slovenly manner, wearing slippers to work. She started neglecting her personal hygiene; she wore soiled blouses and forgot to brush her hair.

Ultimately, Mrs. Chang was diagnosed as having dementia with a superimposed depression. She was treated with an antidepressant medication and became less apathetic and irritable. Her memory and language continued to decline, however, and her confusion worsened. Within two years, she was severely demented. When she became so combative with any change in her routine that even a car ride to her physician's office was an ordeal, her family requested that I take her on as a house call patient.

At our first meeting, Mrs. Chang was sitting in a comfortable armchair in her living room, watching a large-screen television, which was showing *Sesame Street*. She smiled at me and said what sounded like "baba." When I attempted to take her blood pressure, she pushed me away, keeping her arm stiffly bent so as to make it virtually impossible to check the pressure. She said "baba" very loudly and insistently while I tried to listen to her heart, so that the heart sounds were inaudible.

I turned to her caretaker, a devoted young woman who was with her eight hours a day, relieved by either Mrs. Chang's son, her daughter, or an additional paid assistant. I asked how Mrs. Chang spent her day. She had to be cleaned up, dressed, and fed. She was incontinent and drooled and spat quite a bit with the feeding, so the cleaning-up part was repeated several times during the day. She walked from her bed to the bathroom and from there to the living room, where she spent most of her time. Because of her poor balance, her bedroom had been moved to the first-floor guest room. She needed help to walk and usually had to be cajoled to get up at all. Once ensconced in the living room, she watched, or more accurately looked at, television a good part of the day. Periodically she was given some sips of juice, which she appeared to relish. She had a mid-afternoon nap, and on nice days she went out onto the porch. Did she show any evidence of pain or discomfort? No, though she did not like being handled and would have preferred not to get dressed or be bathed. Did she recognize her children? It was not clear that she did. She may have regarded them as familiar, but showed no evidence that she distinguished them from her hired caregiver or from family friends.

Having ascertained that Mrs. Chang was reasonably comfortable and admirably cared for, I cheerfully accepted her as a house call patient. I would check in on her every three months, more often should any new problem arise.

A new problem did arise. One Friday morning, Mrs. Chang's caretaker called to tell me that her charge had a swollen left leg and was unable or unwilling to walk on it. I drove to the house and found Mrs. Chang her usual self, sitting in the living room armchair with the television going. Her left leg was indeed swollen, with the swelling extending from the calf to just above the knee. There was no warmth or redness to suggest infection. There were no bruises or cuts to indicate trauma. The right leg was fine. On further examination, it became clear that the most plausible diagnosis in this sedentary older woman was a deep vein thrombophlebitis (DVT), a blood clot lodged in the veins deep under the surface of the skin.

A DVT—if that was what she had—was a potentially dangerous condition. The clot that was now wedged in a leg vein, causing no more than mild swelling which did not appear to bother Mrs. Chang in the least, could travel to her lungs. Once in the lungs, it would partially block off the circulation, producing shortness of breath, chest pain, and conceivably even death. The conventional treatment was anticoagulation with the medication heparin, administered intravenously, in the hospital. Though I had a strong suspicion that Mrs. Chang's swollen leg was due to a blood clot, I could not be certain without a definitive diagnostic test. And since the other possible diagnoses entailed radically different treatment, I felt I needed to send her to the hospital for a test, but I was very concerned about what would happen to her if I did.

If the test were positive, she would be admitted to the hospital. Once she was in her hospital bed, the intern would write orders for a continuous infusion of intravenous heparin. The intern would also write orders that she was to have her blood drawn daily to determine if the dose of heparin was appropriate and to have her stools checked for blood to make sure the heparin was not causing internal bleeding. She would also undoubtedly have orders for a sleeping pill at night, stool softeners, and a soft diet.

Writing the orders would be easy. Implementing them would be terribly difficult. Mrs. Chang would pull out her intravenous line three times a day, no matter how well it was concealed under layers of gauze, and despite arm restraints on both hands. She would spit and yell when it was restarted or when her blood was drawn. She could not feed herself, so a nurse would have to spend time spoon-feeding her. If the nurse happened to be in the midst of distributing medications or changing dressings or attending to acutely ill patients when the food tray came up, then Mrs. Chang would have to wait. She might have to wait an hour or even two, by which time she would be screaming in frustration. The food, when the nurse got to it, would in all likelihood be cold.

The other patients in Mrs. Chang's room would not take kindly to her screaming. The intern would be asked whether Mrs. Chang could be given a tranquilizer to help her—and her neighbors—calm down. He would accede to this request, and Mrs. Chang would be sedated until the yells subsided. Unfortunately, the amount of medication required to achieve this end would be substantial and might make her so sleepy that she could not stay awake to swallow her food properly. Some of that food, so carefully albeit belatedly ladled into her mouth, would find its way into her lungs instead of her stomach, producing a pneumonia. Mrs. Chang would then be given oxygen and, just when the course of treatment for the deep vein thrombophlebitis was almost completed, would embark on a ten-day regimen of antibiotics for her pneumonia.[35]

Instead of telling Mrs. Chang's children that their mother most likely had a DVT, that she needed to go to the hospital for tests and, if the diagnosis was confirmed, that she would be admitted for treatment, I shared with Mrs. Chang's son and daughter my fears about what would befall her in the hospital. She might, of course, be one of the fortunate ones who tolerated her hospitalization well. If she stayed home with no therapy, she might also be lucky enough to do well. Realistically, neither was very likely. I then told them that there was an alternative: we could treat her at home if she proved to have a DVT.

Home care was a possibility because I could substitute twice daily subcutaneous injections of heparin—injections under the skin—for the standard continuous intravenous drip. I had recently read an article which demonstrated that adequate anticoagulation could be achieved via this route, but which recommended daily blood tests to monitor the dose of the heparin. The risk of complications—either from the underlying DVT or from the heparin—were reported to be the same with the usual hospital-based intravenous therapy approach and with this approach.[36]

Mrs. Chang's family opted to bring her to the hospital for the diagnostic test and if that were positive—which it was—to treat her at home. It took a substantial amount of effort to get everything set up that Friday afternoon. Just finding a pharmacy that stocked heparin for subcutaneous administration in the required doses was a feat. I had to arrange for a visiting nurse to come to the house twice daily to give Mrs. Chang the shots. I had to teach the caretaker and Mrs. Chang's children to look for potential complications.

Mrs. Chang stayed home and received two injections of heparin daily for a week. Her blood was drawn daily for that period. She spent most of that week engaged in her usual routine of washing, being fed, and eyeing the television. Apart from the nurses' visits, her routine was disrupted only in that she walked less and kept her leg elevated more. By the end of the week, I switched her to oral blood thinning medication, and the swelling of her leg had resolved. She required no sedating medications, no arm restraints, and no intravenous needles. She developed no complications.

Another approach would have been to treat Mrs. Chang in an even less technologically intensive manner: with leg elevation and hot packs. A certain proportion of patients with DVT would have gotten better with this treatment alone. A fairly large fraction of those with DVT, however, would not only have failed to improve, but would have developed the chest pain and shortness of breath that are the hallmarks of pulmonary embolism, followed in many cases by death.

The Chang family opted for home treatment with subcutaneous heparin; other families might have chosen hot packs and leg elevation. Crucial to the family's decision making was my explaining to them the hazards of the usual form of treatment and presenting them with other options that offered a reasonable probability of cure. Even the alternative of conservative treatment for her DVT was not tantamount to no treatment; the use of hot packs and leg elevation is a form of treatment. The Chang children regarded this as a bit too conservative and opted for twice daily heparin injections, a treatment that is probably midway between hot packs and hospitalization on the spectrum of medical care. Ideally, the choice they would have been required to make would have been between the various forms of conservative treatment, and not between conventional, maximalist therapy and no treatment at all.

Nadine Chang was fortunate in that she had the material resources and the available family members to care for her at home. Although close to 80 percent of home health care for older people is provided by families rather than through service agencies,[37] contrary to popular conception, families are not always able to handle the increased demands made on them during an acute illness. At 71, Mrs. Chang was relatively young. With increasing age, a rising proportion of individuals need more help than their families or their bank accounts can provide: under 5 percent of the population over 65 is in a nursing home at any given time, but fully 22 percent of those over 85 are in nursing homes,[38] and the lifetime risk of spending time in a nursing home is 30 percent.[39] Of the 1.5 million people in nursing homes in the United States, approximately half, or 750,000, are demented older individuals.[40] For these people, a hospice-style approach to acute illness is just as possible in the nursing home as in the home setting. For them, the nursing home has replaced the home. While the nursing home is seldom as comfortable as a true home environment, it is not lightly abandoned for the unfamiliar terrain of the hospital. If the goal of treatment for a nursing home patient is comfort care, transfer to the acute care hospital can usually be avoided. Provision of care is easier than at home because nursing homes, by definition, already have nursing care on site. Injections, enemas, or oxygen can be readily administered if needed.

Not only can most transfers to hospitals be avoided, but aggressive diagnostic workups and treatment regimens within the nursing home can also be avoided. The questions to be asked when patients become sick are the same whether they are at home, in a hospital, or in a nursing home: How uncomfortable are they? How uncomfortable is the treatment? How likely is it to reverse the acute process? Given that probability, is it worth putting the patients through tests and treatment? To answer those questions, we need to shift our thinking away from the belief that failing to administer the standard treatment is a death sentence for the patient.

We need to accept that a *chance* of recovery is not a sufficient reason to embark on a treatment course if the chance is small, the hazards great, and the patient irreversibly demented. We need to revise upward our standard for what level of chance is enough to pursue a potentially burdensome treatment. Finally, we need to learn more about what these probabilities in fact are—of survival with conventional therapy and of survival without conventional therapy.

❖ 2 ❖
Blessed with Vim and Vigor: The Robust Elderly

Far removed from the world of the demented elderly are the robust elderly. These are the kind of older people we all aspire to be: physically vigorous, mentally acute, a fount of wisdom and experience for their families, busy accomplishing all the things they never previously had the time to undertake. From a medical point of view, the robust elderly are usually not without their share of problems. By age 70 or 80 they often have accumulated a lengthy list of chronic illnesses, ranging from arthritis, the single most common disease in the elderly, to constipation, high blood pressure, diabetes, decreased hearing, glaucoma, and assorted other conditions. Their date books are sprinkled with doctor's appointments; they carry a packet of their medications in their pockets; their night tables are lined with containers for hearing-aids, glasses, and dentures. But despite the diseases, the drugs, and the devices, the robust elderly remain extremely active. They are able to face the challenges of life despite their disabilities. In particular, they are equipped to cope with the stresses of acute illness.

Robust older people, unlike their demented counterparts, have the capacity to understand the nature of new medical difficulties they encounter, whether pneumonia, a heart attack, or cancer. They are able to think about what various proposed treatments would be like for them, and to participate in decisions about their care. They are also susceptible to repeated bouts of illness, as one organ after another comes under siege. As a result, people over 75 account for 5 percent of the total population but 16 percent of hospital discharges and 22 percent of hospital days.[1] Those over 65 represent 11 percent of the population but consume 40 percent of the health care budget.[2] This disproportionate use of health care resources has led economists to ask whether there are any medical treatments which should not be offered to the robust elderly. Are there any medical conditions which should not be treated? Or which should be approached differently solely because of the patient's age? Although policymakers are increasingly interested in such issues, their concerns were far from my mind as I said goodbye to Panos Pappadokoulos.

Sustaining a Lovesick Heart

It was my last day seeing clinic patients as a senior resident in medicine. For three years, as part of my training to be a board-certified internist—during that long period when I had an M.D. degree but was not a full-fledged doctor—I had devoted one afternoon a week to seeing outpatients. Together with my fellow residents, I had been torn away from the demands and the drama of hospital medicine to spend a few hours functioning as a primary care physician: evaluating sore throats, checking blood pressure, monitoring diabetes, addressing family problems. Over the period when I had served as a resident or "house officer," I had built up a small but faithful panel of patients who viewed me as their family doctor.

Panos Pappadokoulos was one of the patients I had known the longest. A spry 87-year-old man, he had had no significant illnesses in his lifetime. I knew a little about him: he had been born in Greece, had come to the United States as a young man, and had worked as a laborer until he was forced to retire at 75 when his employer discovered his true age. He was married, but his wife had advanced Alzheimer's disease. She lived in a nursing home, and he faithfully drove out to visit her each week. He did not think she recognized him. Mr. Pappadokoulos had two daughters who had families and careers of their own. He felt he was an embarrassment to them, with his foreign accent and his old country ways. So he remained proud of their accomplishments at a distance.

There had been no medical reason to schedule an appointment for Mr. Pappadokoulos that June day. I simply wanted to say goodbye to him, to explain to him in person that I was moving on and that another doctor would take my place. Mr. Pappadokoulos, however, had his own agenda. "I want you to check my heart," he told me after we had exchanged the usual pleasantries. "Why—is there something you are worried about?" I wanted to know. He denied chest pain or palpitations or shortness of breath but insisted that he wanted his heart examined. Afterward, I thought, he might explain his concern.

I measured his blood pressure: a healthy 130/70 as usual. I took his pulse and was startled to find that it was 30, less than half his normal rate. Perhaps there was some discrepancy between the true heart rate and the rate discernible from the artery in the wrist. I put on my stethoscope and listened, as I said jokingly, at the source. Still 30. Mr. Pappadokoulos had clear lungs. His mind was as lucid as ever. I told him I needed to do an electrocardiogram (EKG) to get a better understanding of the electrical activity in his heart. He looked anxious. "Is something wrong?" I told him that I was not sure yet, and hooked up the leads of the EKG machine.

There was no longer any uncertainty: Mr. Pappadokoulos was in complete heart block. His normal, biological pacemaker had failed. He was on no medication that might slow his heart so dramatically; he had no acute medical problems that might temporarily cause such a problem. He appeared to have suffered from degenerative changes in his heart which had led to a permanent slowing of his cardiac rate. Implantation of an artificial pacemaker was the only way to prevent the high probability of sudden death.

I told Mr. Pappadokoulos the findings on the electrocardiogram and waited expectantly for him to tell me about symptoms that might have precipitated his request for an examination and that often accompany such a slow heart rate. He shook his head. No, he really had not had any lightheadedness or dizziness or fainting spells. In fact, he had felt quite strong and vigorous. So why had he suspected that he had a heart problem? He had not suspected, he assured me. He had not thought that there were any problems, but he had wanted to make sure because he had found a new lady friend, and he wanted to know just what his heart would permit him to do in her company.

There was a long pause while I gathered my thoughts. How could I explain that there was no medical reason for him to refrain from intimacy with his new friend and at the same time say that he needed a pacemaker? Mr. Pappadokoulos was perplexed. From his point of view, the news that he could benefit from a pacemaker meant that his heart was hopelessly weak—perhaps even weakened by his amorous inclinations. I indicated that there was no causal relationship between his activities (or his fantasies) and the electrical failure in his heart. I told him the heart block was a chance finding, but that insertion of a pacemaker would constitute prudent prophylaxis. "Couldn't I just try without and see how things go?" No, I counseled him. The first warning of impending disaster would in all likelihood itself be catastrophic. At best he would faint, perhaps peacefully in his home with company present to call for help, although possibly while alone at home or while climbing a stepladder to reach the top shelf of his kitchen cabinet. At worst, he would drop dead as his heart slowed so much that it could no longer pump enough blood to his brain to keep him conscious. Or perhaps worse still, he might pass out while driving his car, imperiling others on the road. He was lucky, I pointed out. I just happened to have noticed the inadequate wiring before anything untoward had happened. In fact, I suggested with a half-smile, he owed thanks to his lady friend. She had assuredly not caused the problem, but the fact of her existence and of their incubating relationship had led Mr. Pappadokoulos to request an examination of his heart.

To my surprise, Mr. Pappadokoulos resisted the idea of hospitalization. Was he feeling guilty, thinking he deserved this punishment for infidelity to his demented wife in the nursing home? Was he simply frightened? This determined immigrant had worked all his life, had been in the trenches in World War I, and had survived to age 87 with appendix, tonsils, and gallbladder intact, with no artificial hips or knees and not a single hospitalization to his name. The idea of being an inpatient in a hospital might well terrify him. I decided to enlist the support of his daughters. With his permission, I called his elder daughter, a recently retired high school guidance counselor who was married to a successful businessman.

The contrast between Mr. Pappadokoulos and his daughter, Susan Dinsmore, was striking. He was awkward, a bit untidy and disorganized as he rummaged through the pockets of his baggy pants looking for a slip of crumpled paper with his daughter's telephone number. She was articulate and poised, and immediately began to calculate what appointments she would need to cancel, and who could take her place at various volunteer functions, so she could come to the hospital to join her father. The contrast was even more remarkable in person.

Upon her arrival, Mrs. Dinsmore immediately grasped the medical issues and deluged me with astute questions about the heart problem and the proposed pacemaker. Her father did not even try to follow her line of reasoning as she queried about the risk of side effects, the duration of the hospitalization, and the need for a cardiologist. He alternately stared at his lap and gazed out the window, clearly feeling that this discussion was beyond him. At the end of the conversation, Mrs. Dinsmore turned to her father and told him in a straightforward manner that he needed a pacemaker, that I would make the necessary arrangements, and that he was being admitted to the hospital. When he timidly suggested that maybe a pacemaker was not necessary, or that if he cut all the salt out of his diet he would be fine, his daughter dismissed his theories as mere wishful thinking.

Mr. Pappadokoulos was admitted to the hospital and underwent the uneventful insertion of a permanent pacemaker. He was apprehensive throughout his stay, overwhelmed by the fast pace of the hospital routine—five-minute physician visits, rapid-fire physician-to-physician conversations in unintelligible jargon, X-rays that he was "sent down for" without explanation, and the daily blood-drawing. He remained convinced that he had brought the heart problems upon himself, and unconvinced that he would benefit from what he called the radio in his chest. But he returned home with a heart rate of 60 beats per minute instead of 30, and a good chance of living independently for several years to come.

It was abundantly clear to me and to Mr. Pappadokoulos's daughter that placement of a pacemaker was the right thing to do. Mr. Pappadokoulos was an active, alert, independent man who happened to be 87 years old. He had no other medical problems, and the intervention, while neither cheap nor without risk (the hospital reimbursement by Medicare for a pacemaker insertion in an urban northeastern community teaching hospital in 1990 was $12,000), was relatively safe. The major argument for deciding not to insert a pacemaker is that put forward by those who favor rationing by age. After a certain age (usually defined as around 80), so the argument goes, medical care should be restricted to measures that promote comfort. Medical care designed to prolong life, such as a pacemaker in an asymptomatic individual like Mr. Pappadokoulos, would be prohibited (or at least not paid for by Medicare, the primary medical insurer of the elderly). The basis for such a decision would be the recognition that societal resources are limited, and that the claims on those resources diminish as an individual ages.[3] Society would continue to be obligated to provide comfort care to everyone, regardless of age. The very old—those at least 80, or possibly over 85—would be expected to forgo curative treatment because they had already used up their allotment of medical care and should permit younger generations to receive their full share of life-saving care.[4] A variant on this view is that the very old should forgo life-prolonging treatment because they are already at the end of their lives and if they survive their current illness, they will only go on to succumb to something else, potentially something nastier or more costly, in short order. A final twist on the theme of not-putting-pacemakers-in-87-year-olds is that society's efforts should be in the direction of endowing aging with culturally sanctioned meaning rather than extending life.[5] The goal, as the cliché goes, should be to add life to years and not years to life.

None of these arguments was very persuasive when I was confronted with Mr. Pappadokoulos. From a utilitarian point of view, it was far from clear that leaving Mr. Pappadokoulos in complete heart block would be in the best interest of others. After all, as I suggested, while he might simply die suddenly if his heart slowed further, he might also be afflicted by frequent falls, perhaps fracturing his wrist or his hip. Not only might he require hospitalization because of his fractures; he might need help at home, or he might even have to enter a nursing home if he were sufficiently impaired after the falls. (One study found that 60 percent of elderly patients with hip fractures were discharged from acute care hospitals to nursing homes between 1983 and 1986.)[6] The cost of such palliative care could well exceed the cost of a pacemaker. Moreover, if Mr. Pappadokoulos fainted while at the wheel of his car, he could inflict catastrophic danger on others, as well as on himself. Deciding what treatments are purely life-prolonging in this setting is problematic at best.

As for the argument that if Mr. Pappadokoulos did not die of his heart problem he would soon die of something else, there was no reason to believe that his death was imminent. The life expectancy of an 85-year-old man is now 6.3 years.[7] Is six years an inconsequentially short period of time? It is of course true that Mr. Pappadokoulos might go on to develop Alzheimer's disease and experience a prolonged period of decline. From his point of view, dying suddenly, painlessly, and with all his faculties intact would surely be preferable. But by this argument, perhaps there should be involuntary euthanasia at age 80 in order to guarantee the absence of subsequent debilitating disease. Mr. Pappadokoulos clearly understood that he might die of something more unpleasant later, but he also understood that it was part of the human condition to accept the unpredictable aspects of life and deal with them as best as he could.

Regarding the development of more meaningful roles for the elderly within the surrounding culture, Mr. Pappadokoulos was all for it. He would have been delighted to feel more useful in his community and more valued by his family. But it was far from obvious why he should have to die at a younger age as a price for the realization of this ideal.

The appropriate time to decide not to implant a pacemaker is when a patient's quality of life is so poor that he or his surrogates no longer wish to prolong it, or when he is so ill that his likelihood of surviving a surgical procedure is minimal. Mr. Pappadokoulos had a reasonably good quality of life by his own standards, which is not to say that there was no room for improvement. His incipient romance promised to improve his quality of life further. His economic contribution was minimal: he did continue to consume and hence to contribute indirectly to the economy, but he was no longer productive in the narrow sense of working for a living. From this point of view he was a debit to society, which, after all, paid him a monthly social security check. Clearly, cost-benefit analyses that measure the value of life solely in terms of the economic contribution made by the individual, when applied to the elderly, would never favor intervention on behalf of an elderly person.[8] It is equally true that by any measure of value other than the strictly economic, Mr. Pappadokoulos's life had enormous value. However, even in the absence of this kind of cultural valuation of the elderly, few would deny that an 87-year-old who considers his life worth living has a right to straightforward medical care to maintain that life.

Mr. Pappadokoulos's story is intriguing also because it points to the danger of listening exclusively to the expressed wish of the patient. The prevailing view of medical ethicists is that patient autonomy should be the primary force and often the exclusive factor dictating which medically indicated treatments are undertaken.[9] Mr. Pappadokoulos was mentally intact and in principle able to make decisions about his own welfare. Yet he stated quite clearly that he did not wish to have a pacemaker. When the underlying reason for his refusal was determined, it was evident that Mr. Pappadokoulos held certain beliefs about the cause of his heart problem and its expected future course. He believed that the electrical abnormalities were provoked by what he regarded as illicit or inappropriate involvement with a lady friend, and that they would probably go away if he behaved himself. If they lingered despite irreproachable conduct on his part, he would not discount his theory but instead would conclude that the durability of the problem was suitable punishment for his past indiscretions. Mr. Pappadokoulos understood that physicians interpreted his problem differently, and was able to grasp the fact that I attributed his condition to age-related degeneration of the electrical system of his heart, but he, like many patients, found this inadequate as an explanation.[10] It did not, for instance, explain why the problem had happened to him and not to all 87-year-olds. It did not explain why it had happened now and not six months earlier. Fundamentally, my explanation addressed how heart block occurred rather than why, and it was therefore incomplete and unsatisfactory to him.

Precisely because Mr. Pappadokoulos sought a different kind of theory from the one that was provided, it was impossible to persuade him that his belief system was false. Eliciting the reasons for his seemingly irrational refusal of treatment did not help me alter his conclusion.[11] What did help was the strength of his daughter's conviction that a pacemaker was the correct approach. She prevailed upon him to accept my proffered treatment by telling him that she shared my theory of how this sort of thing worked. She implicitly dismissed his model of health and disease as part of his old-country backwardness and insisted that he accede to my plan. Mr. Pappadokoulos's daughter had a kind of moral authority and persuasiveness that no professional could have.

The vast majority of Americans would, I think, agree that it was right for Mr. Pappadokoulos to get his pacemaker. When polled, most Americans favor decreasing health care costs but do not favor any restrictions on medical care.[12] Even Mr. Pappadokoulos retrospectively agreed. He decided to cut salt and alcohol out of his diet and to pursue his relationship with his lady friend along strictly platonic lines. While he was never entirely certain that it was the pacemaker rather than his personal life-style changes that kept him out of trouble, he regarded the entire episode as a warning to him to change his ways. He came to view the pacemaker as a sort of built-in surveillance device that monitored his behavior.

What if Mr. Pappadokoulos had been 97 instead of 87 when he went into complete heart block? Would I have been as convinced that the pacemaker was warranted? What would his daughter have thought? What about the general public? What if the problem had not been reversible with a fairly simple procedure, but instead had been a malignancy, the treatment of which entailed a major operation?

Surgery in a Nonagenarian

For years I took pleasure in sending first-year medical students to visit Rebecca Landsman at home. Mrs. Landsman was a potent antidote to ageism—the bias against individuals simply because of their advanced age.[13] When I first met her, Mrs. Landsman was a cultured and well-educated woman of 96, endowed with poise, wit, and warmth. Her only significant medical problem was visual loss from macular degeneration, an irreversible process of uncertain eti-ology in which vision is progressively impaired.

Mrs. Landsman lived in an impeccably kept apartment with her 96-year-old husband. She had longstanding ties to the surrounding community, having lived in the area for the entire seventy years of her married life. Her only move was from a single-family house to a two-bedroom apartment at age 94, when she and her husband decided an entire house was excessive for two people; it was too much to maintain and too difficult to negotiate because of the stairs.

Ensconced in her tidy new apartment with a housekeeper to help care for both the apartment and her ailing husband, Mrs. Landsman led a lonely existence. She had outlived her friends and siblings. She had one son, who fortunately lived in the vicinity and came to visit several times a week, but he constituted her entire social life. She felt she could not go out on her own because of her failing eyesight, and for the same reason she could not enjoy theater or even tele-vision. What was even more devastating, she could no longer read books, though she did manage to make out the headlines in a large-print newspaper.

Despite her relative isolation—some of which was self-imposed, since she refused offers of transportation to a senior citizen center and remained steadfastly uninterested in the services of a home companion—she remained in touch with the outside world through the radio, her son, and her housekeeper. She was fascinated with the developments in Eastern Europe in the fall of 1989, com-menting wryly that she had been alive to witness the rise of Com-munism and might yet live to see its fall. She was very much aware of the changing position of women in American society and had strong opinions about issues ranging from sexual promiscuity (bad) to the suitability of pants for women (good).

Mrs. Landsman had remained medically stable for a number of years until, at age 96, she suddenly became weak and fell. She was brought to the hospital where she was found not only to have a broken wrist but also to be profoundly anemic, with evidence of ongoing gastrointestinal bleeding. The wrist was splinted, Mrs. Landsman was given a blood transfusion, and within a day she felt considerably better.

The bleeding, however, did not stop. Every day there were traces of blood in Mrs. Landsman's stools, and on several occasions there were profuse amounts. Mrs. Landsman was reluctant to undergo any tests, feeling that she was 96 and it was time for her to die; she was prepared to do so with good grace. It soon became clear, however, that she would not die with good grace. She would instead become more and more debilitated, more and more dependent on others for even simple tasks like washing herself or dressing. And the process would not take days; it could conceivably take months, or at least weeks, depending on the rapidity of the bleeding. With some reluctance, Mrs. Landsman consented to an upper gastrointestinal series, a relatively simple, painless test involving swallowing liquid barium that would outline the stomach and intestines on an X-ray.

The X-ray revealed a tumor, almost undoubtedly a cancer, in the first part of the large intestine. The appearance of the tumor on the X-ray was so characteristic of a malignancy, and the ongoing bleeding was sufficiently dramatic, that my surgical colleague immediately recommended an operation.

The surgeon was set to go. Mrs. Landsman's son was expecting the surgery to take place. The consulting cancer specialist recommended surgery. Mrs. Landsman was not so sure.

What exactly was the purpose of surgery, she wanted to know. If it was to cure her of a cancer that might kill her, she was not interested. The point of an operation, we agreed, would be to spare her the painful decline in strength and independence that was certain to result if she did not have the surgery. What were the alternatives, she asked. If she did not have the operation, she would almost undoubtedly die, but more to the point, she would do so by a process of slow decline. Her death might not be associated with extreme physical pain, although if she lived long enough for the tumor to grow larger and occlude her intestines, she would experience intense pain. More likely, she would continue to bleed, not profuse amounts, but a steady trickle. As her blood count fell, Mrs. Landsman would become weaker. As she became weaker, she would be at risk of falling, perhaps fracturing another bone as she had when she first developed the bleeding. If she were sufficiently weak, she would be unable to take care of herself. She would suddenly go from being able to dress and bathe herself, from doing her own cooking and merely needing help with shopping and housekeeping, to requiring assistance for her every move. As her blood count dropped, she would also be more prone to developing a heart attack. For while Mrs. Landsman had never experienced chest pain, her electrocardiogram was abnormal, strongly suggesting that she had underlying heart disease. During her usual activities, there was ample blood flow through the narrowed blood vessels supplying oxygen to her heart. If she became profoundly anemic, however, the combination of diminished blood flow to the heart and a lower red blood cell count could result in her heart not getting enough oxygen, even at low levels of activity.

A heart attack might not end matters either. Mrs. Landsman might suffer a non-lethal heart attack that would weaken her further, perhaps leading to her developing fluid in her lungs and feeling short of breath. Or she might go on to develop chest pain from insufficient oxygen to the heart whenever she exerted herself in the slightest.

At some point, her blood count would drop so low that Mrs. Landsman would lead a bed-to-chair existence and would ultimately be bedbound. She would need around-the-clock care, costing as much as $240 a day, or she would have to enter a nursing home. The entire process, from the time of the diagnosis of the tumor to the moment of death, could last months.

Mrs. Landsman thought long and hard about the various options. She had no illusions about her own mortality, and in fact was quite ready to depart from this world. But there was one thing she was quite clear about: she did not wish to be a burden to others, nor did she wish to be dependent on others, which she regarded as equivalent. The prospect of repeated visits to the hospital for transfusions or treatment for chest pain or fractures was dismal. The prospect of fading away over an extended period of time, becoming increasingly dependent, was even more unappealing.

Mrs. Landsman opted for surgery. Ironically, an operation that would probably prove to be curative was performed because it provided the best palliation available. The simplest, most humane, and cheapest way to provide comfort for this very elderly woman was to perform major surgery.

Mrs. Landsman had the operation. She was confused for a few hours afterward because of the effects of the pain medication she received. Otherwise, she had no complications. Two years later she was still living at home. She had had no falls, no chest pain, and no trips to the hospital. Her blood count remained rock-stable. She ultimately died at age 98, at home, in bed, of a stroke. An autopsy showed no signs of recurrent tumor.

Despite Mrs. Landsman's extremely advanced age, she, like Mr. Pappadokoulos, underwent a curative surgical procedure. In her case, the intervention was major by anyone's criteria: she had intra-abdominal surgery, with removal of part of her bowel, under general anesthesia. As with Mr. Pappadokoulos, the patient's family, her physician, and ultimately the patient herself came to see this as entirely appropriate.

The basis for the consensus regarding the reasonableness, indeed the necessity, of proceeding with the surgery was the desire for palliation, for comfort measures. While Mr. Pappadokoulos got his pacemaker primarily to prolong his life (and secondarily to avoid future debilitating accidents or injury to others), Mrs. Landsman had her operation chiefly because it was the only way to make the rest of her life tolerable. The fact that her surgery might be curative—and in fact proved to be—was incidental, practically a side effect of the treatment. The decision to go forward with an operation was made when the physicians, myself as the internist together with the surgeon, discussed Mrs. Landsman's likely trajectory with and without surgery. The main consideration was not length of life; Mrs. Landsman was quite clear that she had no desire to live a great deal longer. In fact she commented that she wasn't at all sure why she was still around, and she regarded her continued presence on earth as faintly ridiculous. Her son reminded her that there were quite a few people who still enjoyed her company, himself and his father among them. My line of argument was that as long as she was here, it was my responsibility to ensure that she be as functional and independent as possible.

It was the prospect of a grim trajectory that persuaded Mrs. Landsman to opt for surgery. She understood that she could die during surgery or in the immediate postoperative period, but she would gladly exchange a quick death for a protracted dying. In fact, palliative treatment without surgery or transfusions was an oxymoron. It was not palliative at all, unless accompanied by active euthanasia. Palliation was far more reliably achieved with surgery than without it. Parenthetically, surgery was probably the cheaper option from both a financial and a psychological point of view. The cost of a single seven-to-ten-day hospital stay was far less than full-time home care. Clearly, for Mrs. Landsman, there was no meaningful distinction between treatment that was strictly palliative and that which was strictly curative.[14]

The discussion that took place among Mrs. Landsman, her son, the surgical consultant, and myself also underlines the importance of considering all the alternatives when making decisions about medical care. The options were not restricted to surgery on the one hand or no treatment on the other. Mrs. Landsman might, for instance, have decided to forgo surgery but to accept careful monitoring of her blood count, with periodic transfusions whenever the count fell below a specified threshold. Although there would still have been a risk of sudden, massive bleeding or of a sufficiently accelerated pace of the bleeding that symptoms such as fainting, falls, or heart problems could have supervened before the drop was detected, it was a risk that Mrs. Landsman might have been willing to take. Her trajectory toward the end of life might then have involved having a blood test every few weeks, with perhaps monthly trips to the hospital for a blood transfusion. Eventually the cancer would have gotten large enough to block completely the passage of stool through the intestine. This would have set up a cycle of vigorous but ineffective contractions, as the bowel vainly attempted to push stool along. Intense pain would have developed, often associated with vomiting. At that point there would again have been choices regarding medical intervention. Mrs. Landsman either could have opted for surgery to relieve the obstruction, or she could have selected a hospice approach: pain medication to be given at home until she died.

The idea of a limited trial of a particular approach also came up in the conversation with the Landsmans. The route that Mrs. Landsman chose—immediate surgery—obviously did not lend itself to a trial; the other, less aggressive approaches did. She might, for example, initially have selected to have transfusions whenever her blood count fell below a specified cutoff. After the third transfusion, she might have concluded that it would make more sense to go ahead and excise the tumor rather than traveling back and forth for transfusions. The concept of a limited trial is only slowly entering common practice.[15] The thinking underlying such trials is that an intervention should be instituted for a specified reason. If it does not succeed in producing the desired result, then it should be discontinued. The widely held belief that stopping treatment is illegal or unethical and is somehow different from failing to start it in the first place does not hold up under philosophical scrutiny.[16] While physicians seem to find stopping treatment psychologically different from not starting it, in fact one can argue that stopping a treatment that is not working should be easier than not starting a treatment that might, after all, prove to be effective.

Mrs. Landsman herself raised the issue of limiting treatment, of following a course other than that which would be the usual approach in a younger person. She contemplated pursuing a less than maximal route because it was clear that she was near the end of her life. At 96, her life expectancy from an actuarial point of view was short. While there is some debate over the maximum expectancy of the human species, most analysts have concluded that if one looks across all societies throughout history, the "natural" life expectancy appears to be about 85 years, plus or minus four,[17] though this may increase to 90 over the next century.[18] Mrs. Landsman was way out at the tail end of the distribution and understood this. There are no good data on the life expectancy at age 96, but as of 1986, there were only 25,000 centenarians in the United States.[19] The overriding goal of medical care for Mrs. Landsman was to keep her comfortable and as independent as possible at the end of her life. How would she have felt had she been twenty years younger, and while still old, not unequivocally at the end of her days?

The robust elderly often do not think of themselves as old. As long as they do not feel old—as long as they are not prevented from walking because of crippling arthritis or severe emphysema, as long as they can perform most of their usual activities—they often do not perceive themselves as different from the way they were a decade ago. They may need to take pills, sometimes large numbers of pills, to keep fluid out of their lungs or to prevent chest pain or control high blood pressure. They may need to wear glasses or a hearing-aid, but they can continue to maintain themselves at home, doing their own cleaning, shopping, and cooking, and they can continue their social lives and sometimes their employment. To ask an intact elderly person to forgo treatment for a potentially reversible illness is and probably should be regarded as unthinkable. This became strikingly apparent in the case of Joseph Kohlman, a vigorous man who had never had any medical problems other than the common cold until he turned 77.

When the Kidneys Fail

Joseph Kohlman lived with his wife in a small apartment. He had two children who lived in the area, as well as an extensive family network. He had retired from his work as a grocer at age 70, though he still occasionally filled in at a local delicatessen. His pension was small, as was his social security check, so he and his wife lived a modest existence. They went to a neighborhood family restaurant for dinner once a week; now and then they went to a movie. For the most part, they spent their time socializing with friends and family, reading the newspaper, and doing household chores. Both Mr. and Mrs. Kohlman were active in their local synagogue and volunteered for assorted projects sponsored by the synagogue.

Mr. Kohlman had been in good health all his life. He needed glasses for reading, as do most people over 50. He had never taken medications on a regular basis and had tended to stay away from doctors until, at age 75, his wife brought him to me for a physical examination. I found that he had markedly elevated blood pressure, and laboratory tests showed a significant impairment of his kidney function. Mr. Kohlman was asymptomatic from both his high blood pressure and his kidney dysfunction, but I was concerned that a narrowing of the blood vessels leading to the kidneys might be responsible for both problems. This could lead to progressive difficulties, which ultimately would produce symptoms: uncontrollable high blood pressure could result in a stroke or a heart attack, and further decline in kidney function would, without dialysis, result in the accumulation of wastes in the blood. This, in turn, would produce fluid retention, anemia, and eventually nausea, dry heaves, confusion, and death.

Mr. Kohlman agreed to come in to the hospital for tests. He had an angiogram, in which dye is injected and X-rays are taken of the arteries leading to the kidneys. He came through the procedure without any problems. The results of the test indicated that one of his kidneys had ceased functioning entirely, and the single blood vessel leading to the other kidney was dangerously narrowed.

Without correction, the already narrowed artery would become even narrower with time, threatening to compromise further the function of the remaining kidney. Mr. Kohlman had two options. He could undergo bypass surgery, in which a synthetic graft would replace the diseased blood vessel, thereby opening up the obstruction and permitting adequate flow of life-sustaining blood to the remaining kidney. He could leave matters alone, hoping that the inevitable decline in kidney function would be slow in coming. A third, theoretical, option was angioplasty, an invasive procedure but one that did not involve general anesthesia or making a major incision—instead, it entailed inserting a tube into the narrow blood vessel and attempting to dilate it by inflating a balloon at the end of the catheter. Unfortunately, because of the diffuse, extensive nature of Mr. Kohlman's atherosclerosis, angioplasty would not be technically feasible. Surgery was a possibility, but because he probably also had atherosclerotic disease in the blood vessels to the brain and the heart, it was deemed very risky. Mr. Kohlman's real choice was between immediate surgery—promising cure but risking a stroke, a heart attack, or even death—or taking a chance with leaving matters as they stood and risking kidney failure in the future.

The Kohlmans debated long and hard with all the physicians involved—myself (the general internist), the kidney specialist, and the heart specialist who had been called in. They talked at length with the vascular surgeon who had been recommended for the operation. The internists focused on the risks of *not* operating: the long-term consequences of rising blood pressure and impaired kidney function. The surgeons concentrated on the risk of *performing* the operation: the real possibility that a man who was currently walking and talking and laughing would in a week be partly paralyzed or unable to speak from a stroke, or would be unable to shave without getting short of breath because his heart had been damaged by a heart attack. The Kohlmans sought a second opinion from another vascular surgeon. Ultimately, they decided that surgery was too risky.

For six months, Mr. Kohlman did relatively well. He saw me monthly, and I made a number of changes in his blood pressure medications. He continued to work part time in the grocery store, to do all the shopping and some of the cleaning at home, and to visit family and friends. His kidney function began slowly to deteriorate. He found that he was not urinating as much as previously, and his lungs began to fill with fluid if he walked a block to the corner store. He became weak and anemic because his kidney was no longer making enough of a hormone critical to the production of red blood cells. Mr. Kohlman received a blood transfusion and felt a little better for a few weeks. Within another six months his single functioning kidney was itself scarcely working. Surgery at that point was too late. I began talking to him about dialysis.

There was no doubt in Mr. Kohlman's mind that he would start dialysis. Much as he regretted that he would have to spend several hours a day, three times a week, hooked up to a machine in a dialysis center, he understood that without dialysis he would die in the near future, and with dialysis he had the possibility of continuing for as long as several years. Joseph Kohlman was a reflective man who did not unthinkingly embrace technological solutions. He had already rejected one invasive procedure, bypass surgery to his kidney. But as long as there was a low-risk treatment for his condition, it simply did not occur to him to opt for anything other than treatment.

The entire Kohlman family—his wife, his siblings, and a multitude of sisters- and brothers-in-law, themselves all between 75 and 85—reacted in the same way to the decision to start dialysis. Perceiving themselves as only a little less vigorous than when they were in their forties, they took it for granted that any fixable medical problem would be fixed. Moreover, dialysis was fully paid for by Medicare, so economic considerations were not an issue. And equally important, because so many Americans have undergone dialysis since Medicare coverage was expanded in 1972 to include this treatment (there are now 91,000 patients per year on dialysis, at a cost of $2.1 billion per year),[20] dialysis has become a household word. It is no longer viewed as a heroic or aggressive or extraordinary therapy by most people. Certainly to the Kohlmans it had become routinized, normalized.

Joseph Kohlman began dialysis as soon as a fistula was created in his arm to facilitate connecting him to a dialysis machine. Neither he nor his wife felt comfortable performing the dialysis at home using peritoneal dialysis, in which a catheter remains in the abdominal cavity, sterile fluid is pumped in, the accumulated wastes enter this fluid and then are pumped out gradually overnight. Instead, he was transported by various relatives three times a week to a dialysis facility, where he was hooked up to a machine alongside ten other patients for two, sometimes four hours, while his blood was filtered of impurities and then returned to his system. He accepted this new facet of his life with equanimity, as he had accepted wearing bifocals and a hearing-aid. It was just one of those things you had to do—unfortunate, distasteful, but necessary. Not to go along with it would be suicidal, Mr. Kohlman felt, and he did not believe in committing suicide. It was his obligation to take what life gave him, the good along with the bad, and to do his best to remain a kind, decent human being, whatever ills befell him. On his days off from dialysis, he went about his business as usual. In fact, life continued in much the same fashion as before dialysis, except that he was always a bit fatigued and decided to give up the grocery store work altogether. His wife gradually took over more and more of the housework, and the relatives visited the Kohlmans more frequently than the Kohlmans visited them. Quietly, insidiously, almost without anyone noticing, Joseph Kohlman was winding down.

Just before his seventy-eighth birthday, a little less than a year after starting dialysis, Mr. Kohlman had a cardiac arrest while on the dialysis machine. Despite the presence at the dialysis center of doctors, nurses, and state-of-the-art equipment, Mr. Kohlman died. His kidney doctor hypothesized that during the dialysis, when there were sudden large shifts of fluid into and out of the circulation, Mr. Kohlman had transiently not received enough oxygen to his heart.

During that critical moment, he was prone to arrhythmias, marked irregularities of his heart rhythm. Because of the underlying poor condition of his heart, it had not been possible to resuscitate him.

Dialysis had clearly not been as unambiguously good a therapy as the Kohlmans had imagined. It was neither as benign in its application nor as unequivocal in its results as, for example, antibiotics for a urinary tract infection. But the Kohlman family had no regrets. They felt that the treatment had provided Mr. Kohlman with a year during which he had been an only slightly paler version of his former self. They were not saddened that he had declined surgery, because that might have meant losing him sooner. They were not dubious about the efficacy of dialysis, since they believed that without it he would have been far more debilitated than he was. They were convinced that dialysis had been the only reasonable option.

The Kohlmans would have been shocked had they known that in England, until recently, dialysis was effectively unavailable to anyone over 55. While there was no explicit prohibition against dialysis for older patients, there was an unwritten rule that those over 55 were ineligible. As a result, 3,000 to 5,000 individuals died of untreated renal failure each year in England.[21] By 1991, the picture had changed substantially: 31 percent of all dialysis patients in England were over 65, though the rate of acceptance of new patients into dialysis programs remains only half that of the United States.[22]

This restrictive standard was enforced by family physicians who routinely informed their patients with chronic renal failure that they would not be accepted by a specialist for further care. One general practitioner explained that patients over 55 are "a bit crumbly" and would not do well on dialysis.[23] In fact, the British decision to limit access to dialysis was an ethical and political decision, not a technical medical one. The experience in the United States, where dialysis is uniformly available, is that dialysis is safe and effective for most older patients. The one-year survival rate for patients aged 65 to 74 receiving dialysis is 77 percent and that for patients over 75 is 69 percent, only slightly lower than the overall one-year survival rate of 85 percent in all patients on dialysis.[24] The risk of complications is associated with the presence of other concurrent medical problems rather than with age.

Not only is dialysis effective in older people, it is also well accepted. Older people generally report a higher degree of satisfaction while on dialysis than their younger counterparts.[25] About half of elderly patients on dialysis report minimal or no decrement in their ability to function while on dialysis. Thus it is difficult to find a basis in fact for the British conviction that patients over 55 simply do not do well on dialysis and therefore should be provided solely with comfort measures.

There are some people in the United States who choose to forgo dialysis. Overall, the statistics reveal that 22 percent of dialysis patients end their lives by terminating the dialysis, and this figure rises to 40 percent in the elderly.[26] Another patient of mine, Matilda Burney, decided at age 88 that she wanted no part of dialysis. Her kidneys were failing, and she understood that dialysis would be potentially life-sustaining. Mrs. Burney was a stoical woman who was fiercely proud of her independence. The prospect of depending on her family to transport her to and from a dialysis center three times a week was intolerable to her. Asking her daughter to perform home dialysis—manipulating a catheter, handling bags and bottles of solutions on a daily basis—was out of the question. When confronted with the likelihood that refusing dialysis would also, ultimately, lead to dependence as she became weaker and confused from the buildup of wastes in her blood, Mrs. Burney simply shrugged. If she reached that point, she said, she would just stay home and be a bother to no one. The reality was a bit different. After six months of progressive kidney decline, Mrs. Burney did indeed become confused. She developed nausea and shortness of breath as her lungs began to fill with the fluid that she was no longer able to eliminate. Honoring her often-stated wish not to be hospitalized, I treated her medically at home. I gave her medication to relieve her nausea and prescribed powerful diuretics to help her failing but still partially functioning kidneys excrete urine. She became homebound and then bedbound. Over the course of a few months, she faded away, increasingly oblivious to her surroundings. She could not be left by herself because of her poor judgment and generally precarious condition, so she required the constant attention of her devoted daughter. She was not, however, aware of how much of a burden she had become. The period of dependence was brief, and Mrs. Burney died at home, quietly.

Panos Pappadokoulos, Rebecca Landsman, Joseph Kohlman, and Matilda Burney were well served by the current system of medical care in America, which offers the elderly all possible medical interventions, with essentially no limits based on age. The major limits arise from technical considerations: there are treatments that are known to carry a very high risk of morbidity or mortality in the elderly. Even here, what is deemed technically inadvisable today may be found quite reasonable tomorrow. For example, it was initially thought that the use of streptokinase, a potent medication that dissolves blood clots in the setting of a heart attack, should be restricted to individuals under 65 because of the inordinate risk of bleeding believed to be associated with this medication in the elderly.[27] Subsequent studies, however, have found that the medication does not actually cause bleeding with any greater frequency in older patients than in younger ones, provided there are no concomitant medical diseases which themselves make bleeding more likely.[28] Similarly, coronary artery bypass surgery was at one time held to be excessively risky in those over 75 or 80.[29] When heart surgeons did use the procedure in selected patients and analyzed the results, they found that even very elderly patients did remarkably well.[30] Thus there may in reality be few if any limitations to care based on lack of efficacy or excessive risk in the robust elderly.

My four patients were well served by the contemporary medical care system in large measure because of the existence of the Medicare program. Medicare, established in 1965 to provide health insurance to those over 65 regardless of need, covers 80 percent of hospital expenses after a deductible of $520 per year.[31] Laboratory and X-ray charges by a hospital are fully covered. Every citizen who qualifies for Social Security benefits is automatically eligible for Medicare Part A at age 65, for no premium whatever. Doctors' bills and outpatient services are covered, also at an 80 percent rate after a deductible is met, if the individual elects to purchase Part B of Medicare. Finally, the 20 percent copayment, along with prescription drugs and other services, can be covered by the purchase of any one of several "medi-gap" insurance policies. In practical terms, most older patients can avail themselves of the full range of medical technology without concern for cost. In particular, Medicare paid almost in full for Panos Pappadokoulos's pacemaker, as it did for Rebecca Landsman's colectomy. Joseph Kohlman's dialysis was paid for in its entirety thanks to the amendment to the Medicare legislation that made dialysis available to all. In fact, perhaps paradoxically, the coverage for less technologically-intensive medical care—medication, for example, or nursing care at home—is far less comprehensive than that for hospital-based care.

The four patients were also well served by the existing system for another reason: they were all mentally intact, and able to express their preferences for how they wished to be treated. The prevailing belief that patients should be fully informed about proposed treatments and any alternatives and should be permitted to decide which treatment they prefer works best when the patient is of sound mind, unimpaired by dementia or depression. Only if patients are capable of understanding information, reasoning using that information, and communicating consistent preferences can they be said to have the capacity to make decisions.[32]

Mr. Pappadokoulos, Mrs. Landsman, Mr. Kohlman, and Mrs. Burney benefited maximally from the existing health care system because the full range of technology was made available to them and they were then able to pick and choose which elements of that technology they deemed desirable. There was little risk of their having medical interventions inflicted upon them or denied them by well-meaning but misguided family members who could only guess their true preferences.

There is one final reason why my four patients, and many others like them, did well with things as they are. All four were functionally intact before they became ill; they were all able to take care of themselves with minimal or no assistance. They could dress, bathe, eat, walk, and get to the bathroom with little difficulty. They were largely although not entirely independent in the other domains crucial for survival—tasks such as shopping, cooking, paying bills, and handling the telephone. This characteristic, more than anything else, rendered them medically indistinguishable from their younger counterparts. Independence in the activities of daily living is far more useful than chronological age in defining for whom conventional medical care, with virtually no restrictions, is medically indicated. The degree of independence in activities of daily living is a powerful predictor of how well a patient will do in an intensive care unit[33] and of whether a person will survive a cardiopulmonary arrest.[34] The capacity for self-maintenance appears to be a more reliable marker than any physiological parameter, such as kidney function or exercise capacity, of where a person stands on the trajectory of life. And that, for most people, is crucially important to making any decision to limit medical care. It is not merely a matter of personal preferences for home versus hospital care, surgery versus medical approaches, or chemotherapy versus radiotherapy. Nor is it merely a matter of the technical advantages of the competing forms of care. Values, the extent to which individuals are risk-averse, and medical facts all play a role in shaping decisions to limit care. But perhaps paramount in significance is the assessment made by physicians as to whether a patient is gradually inching along on the road from birth to death, or whether he is plunging down a sharp descent, relentlessly headed toward his demise.

❖ 3 ❖

Facing the Final Days: The Dying Elderly

At the other end of the spectrum from the robust elderly are the dying elderly. The dying are not merely in the last stage of the life cycle; they are at the very end of their lives. Decisions about medical care can affect the quality of their remaining time and can determine the manner of their death, but cannot ultimately affect their fate.

More than any other segment of the elderly population, the plight of the dying has attracted public attention. We have been treated to the specter of hopelessly ill patients who do their dying in an intensive care unit, rendered mute by an endotracheal tube, visited by family members for brief ten-minute periods that are wedged in between invasive procedures. They die after lying helplessly in a world of perpetual daylight, where time is marked by the rhythmic sighs of the ventilator and the beeps of the cardiac monitor.[1] We read about patients who are subjected to aggressive, painful, and unwanted treatment, apparently at the behest of physicians who refuse to give up or courts which uphold an overriding interest in the preservation of life or, occasionally, families who cannot let go. Fear of precisely this kind of protracted, meaningless dying has stimulated interest in advance directives. It has led some sufferers from terminal illness to seek the assistance of Dr. Jack Kevorkian, a retired pathologist who has made it his mission to put patients out of their misery by use of a suicide machine or, in most cases, inhaled carbon monoxide gas administered in Kevorkian's van.[2]

These grim portrayals have also helped to generate a growing consensus about what constitutes a good death. The new image of the good death bears a striking resemblance to that of an earlier age, before the locus of death moved from the home to the hospital[3] and before the triumph of individual self-determination—over all facets of life, including dying—as a transcendent societal value.[4] The good death is peaceful, painless, and takes place at home, with loving family in attendance.[5] It comes quickly, without a preceding period of debility and dependence. The role of the physician in caring for a dying patient, in this model, is to usher in the good death by eliminating the distressing manifestations of the dying process—shortness of breath, vomiting, or pain.

As a geriatrician, I expected that I would watch many of my patients enter the realm of the dying. Old age, after all, is not a condition that anyone survives. I knew that my role would sometimes be to cure my patients, sometimes to restore them to a tolerable level of functioning, and often to maintain their comfort as they sickened and died. There would, of course, be a number of obstacles to enabling patients to die a good death. Some patients might not want to accept their destiny without a struggle. They might choose to rail and storm against their diagnosis, adamant that they would not go gentle into that good night, insistent that I do everything possible to eke out a few more moments of life. Should they be denied technological interventions that offer a small chance for a brief prolongation of life, even if this is a course they desperately wish to pursue? Would we react differently to such a plea if the treatment requested were extremely expensive? If the patient were willing to pay for it, regardless of cost, out of pocket? Other patients might have quite the opposite response to the news of their imminent death. Instead of trying to prolong their lives, they might seek to get it all over with as quickly as possible. Rather than place themselves at the mercy of their disease, they might choose to seize control over their fate in the only manner remaining to them: by actively ending their own lives. If such patients requested my help in committing suicide, would I oblige them? Should I?

I have come to realize with considerable chagrin that a major difficulty in providing medical care to facilitate a good death is that it is not always clear just when the dying process has begun.

Determining When Dying Starts

I first met Jennie Rosetti when she was an inpatient, hospitalized with a small stroke. She was a vivacious 85-year-old who had not seen a doctor in twenty years because she had been unambiguously healthy. I was assigned to her care as part of my responsibilities as a hospital staff physician.

Jennie had been admitted in the evening after she noticed that her left arm and leg did not seem to work properly. I learned from the emergency room record that she had been brought in by a friend; she had been evaluated and thought to have had a stroke. I found Jennie—that is how she asked me to address her—sitting in bed polishing off her breakfast. I introduced myself and asked her to tell me what had happened to her. "I kept dropping my fork last night," she told me. "Now I'm doing okay because I'm putting my fork in my right hand. Yesterday I figured I better stop eating and I went to get up from the kitchen table." She smiled at me and added, by way of explanation, "I live alone in a one-bedroom. It's a third floor walk-up with an eat-in kitchen." Then she resumed her tale. "My left leg was a dead weight. I managed a few steps and then realized I was not going to be able to make it the twenty feet to the living room. I grabbed onto the sink with my right hand, leaning hard against the cabinet under the sink. I figured my arm and leg had fallen asleep from sitting too long in one position, though I had to admit this was quite a deep sleep." She smiled again, as though to acknowledge it sounded a bit preposterous. "I waited a while and then tried to shake my left arm. I could move it only very slowly. I stood there and thought to myself, *I'm having a stroke.*"

This was a rather detailed account of the history; but I decided to let Jennie continue a bit longer. "I tried to figure out how I could reach the telephone. It was really only a few feet away on the coffee table, but there was nothing but open space between me and the telephone—nothing sturdy to grab onto. I waited a while longer, thinking perhaps the weakness would pass. Instead, it seemed to get worse, and I realized my left leg was about to give way beneath me. So I slid down to the floor and started to crawl. I slithered across the smooth kitchen floor—I must have looked like I was doing the sidestroke on land, dragging my left side. Maneuvering across the rug and around the corner was trickier. I'm not sure how long it took to reach the telephone—maybe half an hour, maybe longer. I propped myself up against the sofa, my legs straight out in front of me under the coffee table, and dialed my good friend Barbara, who lives down the street." She paused for a moment, but before I could get a word in, plunged on with her saga.

"I must have looked awfully funny, crawling along. I wish someone could have seen me and taken a picture. I guess I looked kind of comical wedged in between the sofa and the table, too, but Barbara didn't think so when she came in. Thank goodness I'd given her a key," Jennie rambled on. "Actually, I had given it to her so she could water the plants when I went away for the weekend, and forgot to get it back from her. That was a month ago," she added parenthetically, to make sure I was following the story. "I told Barbara I was eating Japanese style—you know, on the floor. My son had been in Japan during the War. He told me all about things like that. Of course he never had a chance to eat in a Japanese home. They were the Enemy then. But my son never really believed the Japanese were bad people. It was just their government. Like today . . ."

I could tell there was nothing wrong with Jennie's speech. Often a stroke that affects the left side of the body, while sparing the language center of the brain, can produce slurred speech. Her speech was perfectly clear. Moreover, I could tell this feisty lady was mentally intact and, before last night, had evidently been physically intact. "How are you this morning?" I asked, trying to bring her back to the present.

"I'm a little better," she said, and began demonstrating just how much movement she had in her left arm. "And look at this!" She pulled the bedclothes off her legs and began to raise her left leg off the bed. She could only raise it an inch or two and then it fell back down. She grinned at me. "I keep lifting it a little bit, five times every hour. I had a friend who had a stroke, and he had a physical therapist, and she gave him exercises—"

I interrupted her again to assure her that she, too, would receive physical therapy. But right now I needed to figure out why she had had a stroke; I needed to make sure she had not had a heart attack in addition; then she could proceed full steam ahead with rehabilitation.

Jennie was so determined and so energetic that she was discharged to a rehabilitation hospital within three days. She had not had a heart attack, but she had an irregular heartbeat which almost undoubtedly had led to a blood clot traveling to the brain. She was given an anticoagulant to prevent further blood clots after an unsuccessful attempt to convert her heart rhythm electrically to a regular beat. Her strength improved daily; by the time of the transfer to the rehabilitation hospital, she could already stand and take a few steps with a walker.

I saw Jennie in my office two months later, shortly after she had returned home. She pranced into the office wearing bright pink slacks and jogging shoes, waving a cane mischievously. "I use this for protection," she told me. "Just to make sure nobody will take advantage of an old lady like me." Jennie really did need the cane, and not just for self-defense. She had quite a bit of difficulty making it up and down the stairs to her apartment. Her friend Barbara wanted her to move in with her for a while, and her son, who had flown in for a week, wanted Jennie at least to move to a first-floor apartment. Jennie was stubborn: she wanted to stay where she had lived since the death of her husband ten years earlier. She had friends in the neighborhood, and she was in walking distance of a small shopping area. She did not want outside help either, help from an agency that provided homemakers (to assist with housekeeping and shopping) and home health aides (to help with personal care such as bathing). "I can manage," Jennie asserted. "And if I can't manage anymore, I don't want to be around."

She did manage, initially husbanding her strength for an excursion outside only once a week. Six months later she could go up and down the stairs with minimal difficulty, and truly no longer needed the cane. She bounded into my office, bubbling over with the details of her upcoming day trip with a senior citizens' club to which she belonged. "Who knows? I might even find myself a boyfriend," she told me. "I think I look pretty good, don't you? I just had my hair done and I don't think anyone would know I'd had a stroke." I agreed—she really did look terrific. "But you know," she added, "I saw a lot of people in that rehab hospital who were in awful shape. There was one lady who couldn't talk at all. Only seventy years old. Every time she tried to say something and the words wouldn't come out, tears came to her eyes. And there was a man who had weakness on the left side, like me. They thought he would get better, but he didn't. They worked on him every day but he never got any better. His wife wanted to take him home but his children didn't think she could take care of him. They thought he should go to a nursing home." Jennie shook her head soberly. "If I can't take care of myself, what's the point? I don't want to be a burden to anyone."

I listened and asked whether her son and her friend Barbara knew how she felt. "They know," she told me. "They don't like it, but they know." We talked about designating a health care proxy, someone who could make decisions on her behalf should she become critically ill and unable to make health care decisions for herself. "But you still have quite a lot of spunk left," I commented as she trotted off.

The next time I saw Jennie was three months later, in the hospital intensive care unit. She was on a respirator, with an arterial catheter in place to permit constant measurement of blood pressure and oxygen content, a catheter in her bladder to determine how much urine she excreted, an intravenous line threaded through a large vein in her neck, and a nasogastric tube for feeding. Barbara told me that Jennie had been sick for a few days with what she thought was the flu. She had had a bit of a fever, a slight cough, nothing dramatic. Barbara had gone to visit her family for the weekend. She had called Jennie when she got back Sunday evening and was dismayed that no one answered the phone. Jennie almost never went out in the evenings, and it was a cold January night. Fully expecting to find Jennie sitting on the floor, cheerfully awaiting rescue, Barbara went into the dark apartment. Jennie was slumped over in an armchair, breathing rapidly, her face flushed. Barbara called to her, shook her gently, yelled in her ear, but she could not wake her up. This time it was not a stroke. It was overwhelming pneumonia, involving three of the five lobes of her lungs.

For the next three days, Jennie received respirator support to breathe for her, intravenous antibiotics to fight the infection in her lungs, and artificial hydration and nutrition to sustain her while the fight continued. Her temperature came down and her white blood cell count fell to the normal range, but she continued to depend on the respirator for oxygen. She was no longer unconscious, as she had been on admission, but she could not speak because she remained attached to the ventilator. When I asked her to squeeze my hand, she did. She could answer yes/no questions by nodding or shaking her head. She winced with pain whenever her blood was drawn. When the nurses suctioned sputum from her lungs, Jennie tried to push them away. Her hands were restrained to prevent her pulling out her various tubes and lines. Whenever I came to examine her, she looked at me imploringly, beseechingly, sometimes accusingly. I told her that she had pneumonia and was getting anti-biotics. I explained that she was on a breathing machine because she was unable to breathe for herself. I told her that I hoped her lungs would improve and we could get her off the machine soon. She closed her eyes and turned away.

On the fourth day, Jennie's blood pressure began to drop and her kidneys began to fail. She became more and more lethargic, and gradually drifted into unconsciousness. I sat down with Jim Rosetti, Jennie's son, and her faithful friend Barbara, to discuss the options.

My overwhelming impression was that Jennie Rosetti was dying. However, I could not give the odds that she would come through this. There simply were no good data on the likelihood of survival of 85-year-old women with underlying atrial fibrillation and a history of stroke who had trilobar pneumonia and failed to respond to appropriate antibiotic therapy. I could tell them that some people hospitalized in her condition recovered totally, much as Jennie had after the stroke. I could also tell them that a great many elderly people who came in as sick as Jennie had been and who began to develop complications as she had were headed for an inexorable decline: one calamity would occur after another, ultimately eventuating in death. We talked about the choices: we could give her a potent medication to maintain her blood pressure; if the kidney function deteriorated further we could dialyze her. There could be more troubles in the offing: she might go on to have a heart attack; she might develop gangrene of the intestines if the low blood pressure led to inadequate blood flow to the intestines; she might get a stress ulcer, leading to massive internal hemorrhage. My concern was no longer with her suffering—she was beyond the point of being able to experience pain—but rather whether she had any reasonable chance of surviving this devastating illness and resuming the independent life she so prized. I thought it more likely that she was on a relentless downhill course which could be slowed but not stopped.

We all agreed that Jennie would not want to live with brain

damage that rendered her unable to communicate or recognize her friends and family. She had stated quite explicitly that she did not wish to live if she were mentally alert but totally dependent on others for survival. We also agreed that Jennie would have regarded a prolonged period on a respirator, unconscious, as an offense to human dignity. Barbara related a conversation she had had with Jennie on the subject of Karen Quinlan, some years before. "They talk about the sanctity of life!" Jennie had said. "What about the sanctity of death? When someone has died, is it right to pretend they're alive and do all kinds of things to them? That Karen Quinlan—she can't breathe on her own, she can't eat on her own, she can't communicate or recognize anyone. I guess they can't say she's dead until her heart stops. So they should put her to bed and leave her in peace. Technically maybe she isn't dead but she sure is gone. They should have some respect for goners just like for dead people." Our problem, of course, was to be sure that Jennie was really a "goner" before we decided to give up on her.

Knowing that Jennie did not want a death preceded by a long period of invasive procedures, we chose to wait another forty-eight hours. During that time, she would receive intravenous medications to maintain her blood pressure, and she would continue to get antibiotics. We would monitor her kidney function. If she was improving after two more days of treatment—if she woke up and her kidney function stabilized and her lung condition improved— we would press on with treatment. If not, we would conclude that the life-sustaining medical interventions had been unsuccessful and discontinue them.

It was a harrowing two days. The nursing staff in the intensive care unit were all rooting for Jennie. I was worried that she would neither get better nor get worse; instead she would remain unchanged and we would not know whether she was dying despite everything or whether she might yet improve. On the second night after our family conference, it became clear that all of Jennie's organs, one after another, were falling apart. Her liver function tests, a measure of damage to the liver, showed massively elevated liver enzymes, consistent with shock liver, or profound damage due to lack of blood flow. Her heartbeat, which had been rock-steady throughout her illness, again became irregular as it had been at the time of her stroke. An electrocardiogram indicated that this time the atrial fibrillation was a complication of a major heart attack.

At two in the morning, when the blood pressure began to drop again despite the continued use of the blood-pressure-raising medications, I called Barbara and Jennie's son to apprise them of the latest developments. They both came in to see her. They sat with her, they held her hand, and they cried. Then they asked that she be given no further medications and have no more intravenous lines or tubes placed. They decided for the time being to leave in place whatever tubes were already present, just in case the manipulation involved in removing them could produce discomfort. They sat quietly in the waiting room for a few minutes. Just as they got up to go home, having said their goodbyes, the nurse came out to tell them that Jennie had died.

Stopping life-sustaining treatment for Jennie Rosetti had been relatively easy. It had been sad to lose her, but the medical team had had strong evidence that further therapy would have been futile, and Jennie herself had given reasonably clear indications of her preferences regarding care at the end of life.

A major medical challenge in taking care of Jennie in the intensive care unit (ICU) had been to try to determine whether she was dying. Much of the furor about the high cost of medical care in the last six months of life[6] and about the allegedly overly aggressive treatment of dying patients[7] hinges on the assumption that it is possible to predict who is going to die. A variety of tools have been developed to help predict outcomes of treatment in the very sick elderly, but until extensive data from multiple ICUs nationwide have been collected and analyzed, it will remain very difficult to make accurate predictions, taking into account the specific situation of a given patient.[8]

Even if precise predictions in general remain a goal for the future, there may be certain circumstances in which particular treatments can be said to be futile. Unfortunately, the concept of futility has also proved elusive.[9] Clearly, physicians are under no ethical or legal obligation to provide treatment that is not, by prevailing standards of care, medically indicated: professional standards dictate that doctors should not treat the common cold with penicillin or cancer with laetrile, regardless of what patients request.[10] Less clear is the obligation of physicians to provide treatment that in principle is rational—for instance, cardiopulmonary resuscitation for sudden death—but that in the particular situation of a given patient is extremely unlikely to produce the desired outcome. The recognition that elderly patients residing in nursing homes virtually never survive attempted cardiopulmonary resuscitation has led to the suggestion that doctors withhold this treatment.[11] The concept of futility presumed by this approach has been further refined and extended to treatments other than CPR: some authors have proposed that physicians regard a treatment as futile if in the last 100 cases it has been unsuccessful.[12] The difficulty with this seemingly straightforward definition is that it hinges on what constitutes being unsuccessful, which in turn depends upon the goal of therapy. If the goal of a ventilator is to avoid death, then it succeeds in its goal even if all it does is maintain a patient in a permanent state of unconsciousness. If the goal of treatment, on the other hand, is to restore a person to his previous state of functioning, then a ventilator that maintains a patient in a vegetative existence is a failure.

Since I could not be sure that Jennie Rosetti was dying, but neither did I wish to embark on a protracted course of invasive therapy only to fail in the end, I proposed a limited trial of treatment. Jennie's son, her friend, and I agreed to use the full range of medical technology to combat the pneumonia for two days. If, after that time, she had not improved in terms of her pulmonary condition and her mental status, I would discontinue the treatment that had not worked.

It could, of course, be argued that stopping treatment after a fixed period of time if it had not achieved its ends was highly arbitrary. Just because Jennie had not woken up after two days did not prove that she would not wake up in five days. If she remained ventilator-dependent after forty-eight hours, she might nonetheless be able to be weaned from the machine a week later, once she had recovered from the heart attack she had suffered in the interim. Just how reasonable it is to test medical therapy empirically for a limited period depends, once again, on how certain you wish to be that the therapy truly is ineffective. There is some suggestion that the majority of patients and their families are willing to undergo a great deal for a small reward. Studies of the preferences of survivors of intensive care units have consistently found that the majority would favor undergoing intensive care again, even if it prolonged life by as little as a month.[13] The trouble with such studies is that patients who have survived one encounter with critical illness have a tendency to overestimate their probability of surviving in the future: they will quite naturally tend to think that although the risk to the population as a whole may be 50 percent or even 10 percent, their personal risk is much closer to zero since they already demonstrated the capacity to survive. Even family members of individuals who died in an ICU tend to be overly optimistic; they may use magical thinking to revise downward the odds of dying with which they are presented, reasoning that the general statistics somehow do not apply to them.[14] If instead of being told that they had a 10 or 20 percent chance of survival with ICU care, patients were told they had an 80 to 90 percent chance of dying with ICU treatment, and a 99 percent chance of dying without it, and that 90 percent of the time the only difference between the two situations was that in one case they would die quickly and quietly, and in the other they would die after weeks of poking and prodding, how many would in fact choose the ICU?

Jennie Rosetti had given some indirect indications of what was important to her: she had made it quite clear that she did not want to live if she was dependent on others. In her comments about

Karen Quinlan, the young woman in a coma whose parents had fought to have her respirator removed, she had been adamant that she regarded life in a persistent vegetative state as no life at all. Moreover, she viewed continued medical treatment of such individuals as profoundly disrespectful. In the days before she herself lapsed into coma, she appeared to have been communicating that she had had enough, that she was convinced she was dying and did not want more to be done—but that was my subjective interpretation. And she most definitely had not addressed the issue of the level of certainty she considered necessary before she would authorize withdrawal of life-sustaining treatment.

Courts of law have not been particularly helpful in this area. Since competent patients have the right to refuse life-sustaining treatment, judges have reasoned that incompetent patients should not be compelled to undergo treatment. At first, the withdrawal of life-sustaining treatment was limited to patients who were terminally ill. This has been extended, with the case of Karen Quinlan, to patients in a persistent vegetative state. With Nancy Cruzan, another young woman in a persistent vegetative state after suffering brain damage in a car accident, the Supreme Court argued that all life-sustaining medical treatment—whether respirators or artificial nutrition—could be withheld.[15] Thus, patients who are "incurably and critically ill" may have life-sustaining treatment withdrawn if there is sufficient evidence that that is what they would have wanted or, in most states, if the burdens of treatment outweigh the benefits. The problem with Jennie was that it was not clear whether she was incurable—though with each passing day, her prognosis was poorer; the evidence about what she would have wanted was suggestive but hardly definitive; and once she had become comatose, it was hard to argue that there were any burdens to her of continued treatment. Ultimately, the decision made by Barbara, Jim, and myself to limit further treatment was based on what we considered a reasonable approach—consistent, to be sure, with Jennie's previously stated wishes, but hardly a direct corollary of her thinking.[16]

Fortunately, determining when dying starts is not regularly as difficult as with Jennie Rosetti. Experienced physicians can usually ascertain, with a fairly high level of confidence, when the end is beginning. But once the line has been crossed, the path to a peaceful death is still far from secure. Patients, rather than embracing a course of palliation, may respond to the victory that mortality is about to proclaim with one last attempt to control their fate. Often, this takes the form of expecting physicians to combat their illness with all the weapons in their medical armamentarium: chemotherapy for the patient with widely metastatic cancer, a ventilator for the person with respiratory failure, cardiopulmonary resuscitation for the individual whose heart has stopped. Occasionally, this final manifestation of the passionate desire for self-determination takes the form of suicide, with or without the assistance of a physician.

A Cry for Help

Without a doubt, Mrs. Renan was one of the most challenging patients I have taken care of. She came to see me for the first time at age 90, not having seen a doctor in years. She chose me because I specialized in elderly people and my office was in walking distance from her apartment. The first visit focused principally on her philosophy of medical care and mine, so we could assess whether we were a match.

Mrs. Renan's overriding concerns were that she be kept comfortable in the event that she became acutely ill, and that her life not be prolonged by technological means. Although she was still a vibrant woman who lived alone and did most of her own cooking, cleaning, and shopping, she felt her life was drawing to a close. When the curtain rose on the final act, she felt, there was no sense in delaying the denouement. Moreover, though I found her an engaging, mentally intact person in reasonably good physical health apart from modest hypertension, Mrs. Renan stressed that she could no longer do many of the things that gave life meaning to her. Her eyesight was impaired and could not be improved upon, limiting her ability to read. Her hearing was failing despite bilateral hearing-aids, so she could no longer appreciate music. She enjoyed the attention of her daughter, son-in-law, and a loyal elderly friend, but was afraid of becoming burdensome to those she loved if she lost any further functioning. She felt that medical interventions that prolonged life at the cost of progressive disability were strenuously to be avoided. I agreed that I would discuss all treatment options with her, and I told her I supported her wish that her medical care have as its goal comfort and dignity. She signed me on.

I saw Mrs. Renan from time to time over the next year. She developed painful osteoarthritis, the wear-and-tear arthritis that afflicts most older people to some degree or another sooner or later. Mrs. Renan's knee and hip pain threatened to diminish her mobility and increase her dependence, precisely what she feared most. Ultimately, the arthritis became tolerable with medication. Mrs. Renan adamantly refused to take antihypertensive medication, despite my argument that she was placing herself at increased risk of a stroke, which could make her totally dependent on others.

On a follow-up visit to assess the efficacy of the arthritis medication, Mrs. Renan reluctantly disclosed that she had been having rectal bleeding. Every time she moved her bowels, she noted bright red blood in the toilet bowl. She did not have bleeding only when she wiped herself: sometimes she noticed a few drops of blood staining her underwear even when she did not move her bowels. I had been concerned about the possibility of gastrointestinal bleeding induced by the arthritis medication and had urged her to be alert for abdominal symptoms in general and black stools in particular. During the course of the physical examination that Mrs. Renan grudgingly allowed me to perform, I found a rock-hard, nodular, bleeding mass at the opening of the rectum.

The bleeding was not from an ulcer or gastritis induced by the arthritis medication. The bleeding was almost certainly from a cancer of the rectum.

Mrs. Renan was nonplussed. She was, after all, fully expecting to die in the near future. She had been convinced even before the appearance of her tumor that she was in the final stage of her life. Her concern, given this new development, was with envisioning the future—what remained of it. I described the various options. Curative therapy would entail major surgery: she would need an abdomino-perineal resection in which the rectum itself is removed and the intestines are diverted through the skin via a colostomy for purposes of evacuation. That, Mrs. Renan said, was absolutely out of the question. Radiation therapy, I told her after consultation with a radiotherapist, would involve daily visits to the hospital for several weeks, was unlikely to achieve much, and was very likely to be associated with significant side effects such as radiation proctitis, an inflammatory condition that results in pain and diarrhea. The only alternative Mrs. Renan found acceptable was to leave the tumor alone.

Over the next few months, the cancer produced no physical symptoms. The principal development was that Mrs. Renan began to dwell almost exclusively on her death: she talked about it, she waited for it, she despaired that it had not yet arrived. She lost even her previously attenuated capacity to enjoy life. She ate little and slept poorly, always worrying that blood might stain her nightgown or sheets. Mrs. Renan met the criteria for a clinical depression, but she refused antidepressant medication and was opposed to seeing a psychiatrist. Since she was not overtly suicidal, nor was she endangering anyone else, I could not compel her to accept treatment of her depression. She remained at home, mired in gloom.

When the physical symptoms escalated, they were of two varieties. First, Mrs. Renan developed intermittent incontinence. The tumor impeded the normal function of the anal sphincter and partially obstructed outflow from the rectum. When Mrs. Renan became constipated—which occurred often, especially with her poor diet and minimal exercise—she suffered from excruciating pain as she tried to pass a hard stool beyond the constricting tumor mass. When she used even the mildest laxative, she quickly developed loose, sometimes watery stools, which tended to flow out before she could reach the bathroom.

Claire Renan had always been a dignified woman, and finding that she was unable to prevent herself from soiling her underwear was a profound assault on her dignity. Having to depend on her daughter for shopping was bad enough; hiring a housekeeper to clean once a week had struck a blow to her self-sufficiency; but wearing a diaper at night was supremely humiliating. Ultimately, her difficulty in maintaining personal hygiene was so great that she required a live-in companion who was available to help her get to the bathroom and wash up. Between her arthritis, which limited her mobility, her impaired vision, which was responsible for a series of miscalculations about just where the toilet was, and the unpredictable behavior of her bowels, Mrs. Renan felt she no longer had control of even her most basic bodily functions. I tried Mrs. Renan on a low dose of a tranquilizing medication in an effort to help her deal with her overwhelming anxiety as she lost control of her physical self. The medication made her mind feel fuzzy, exacerbating rather than alleviating the problem by making her feel that she was losing her mind as well as her body.

To compound matters, the gradual loss of blood resulted in progressive weakness. Mrs. Renan did not have the energy to do much more than sit up in bed. She found it increasingly difficult to walk around even within the confines of her apartment. I felt I could do something about the weakness: the lack of strength derived quite simply from lack of blood, which could be remedied by means of a blood transfusion. It would be entirely in keeping with our agreed-upon goal of keeping Mrs. Renan as comfortable as possible to bring her over to the hospital for several hours in order to administer a transfusion.

Mrs. Renan protested vehemently. She would accept no intervention such as a blood transfusion which had the potential to prolong her life, no matter how much transient relief of discomfort it offered. The tumor was still relatively small and would take quite some time until it had grown enough to produce a fatal bowel obstruction. There was no evidence that it had spread to other parts of her body such as the liver, so an imminent death from metastases was also unlikely. The only way that the tumor could kill her in the near future was if it produced copious enough bleeding that she no longer had a sufficient blood supply to nourish her vital organs—heart, kidneys, and brain. Mrs. Renan was determined to die and was adamant that if the only way she could do so was to bleed to death, then she would bleed to death. I could make things a great deal easier, she suggested, by facilitating her death with medication. I told her I had treatment to ease her suffering, in this case a transfusion. She shook her head. If I thought a transfusion would ease her pain, I simply did not understand. As long as she remained conscious, she would suffer. The only relief for her suffering was oblivion, preferably permanent, irreversible oblivion.

At this point I insisted that I needed the assistance of a psychiatrist to care for Mrs. Renan. Together, the psychiatrist and I persuaded her to take an antidepressant medication. After multiple trials, we hit upon a medication that she was able to tolerate without exacerbating her constipation and without precipitating jitteriness. Unfortunately, while the medication helped Mrs. Renan sleep through the night, it did little to alter her mood. I felt that consideration should be given to the use of electric shock therapy, which sometimes produces dramatic results when antidepressant medication either fails or has unacceptable side effects. However, both the initial psychiatrist and another psychiatrist called in for a second opinion felt that Mrs. Renan was not a candidate for shock treatment. They believed that she was not truly depressed, but rather was reacting logically, albeit dramatically, to what was, for her, an unendurable existence.

As Mrs. Renan became weaker, she became even less able to care for herself. When she declined to the point at which she led a bed-to-chair existence and needed help with bathing, dressing, and even eating, she agreed to enter a nursing home. She no longer derived pleasure from being in her own home since her home had been converted to a miniature hospital: she had a hospital bed, she had a commode in her room so she did not have to go to the bathroom, and she had a buzzer to summon her personal care attendant. She almost never stepped out into her living room, with its magnificent river view; she seldom looked at the books in her library; and she rarely ventured into the kitchen where she had prepared meals for nearly fifty years. The benefits of remaining at home were minimal; in fact, she found the familiar environment a constant reminder of the person she used to be and was no longer.

When Mrs. Renan entered the nursing home, she took to bed. She effectively gave up on her body, which had proved so fickle and feeble, and became totally passive in her personal care. She began to eat less and less and to sleep more and more. She continued to refuse blood tests and antihypertensive medication, accepting only the antidepressant, which she used as a sleeping pill, and narcotics against pain. When she was awake, she asked incessantly when the end would come. She accused me of abandoning her because I said I would not and could not give her a lethal injection. She inveighed against the staff at the nursing home for being insufficiently caring because nothing they did relieved her suffering. Even when she slept, she looked angry. When she finally died, after months of gradual blood loss and minimal nourishment, she had a peaceful expression on her face.

What made Claire Renan such a troubling patient to take care of is that she systematically rejected the medical care I offered her. We had agreed on the goal of treatment: Claire's comfort. What I had not bargained for was that she would regard as inadequate all the comfort measures I proposed, and demand instead euthanasia.

The technical phrase for what Claire Renan wanted is "physician-assisted suicide" or "physician aid in dying."[17] She did not, after all, request that I shoot her or push her out of the nursing home window. Rather, she expected me to use equipment within the medical armamentarium toward a lethal end. She did not even request until close to the end that I give her a lethal injection. Claire would have been quite satisfied had I prescribed a large quantity of a sedative or narcotic and instructed her on how many to take in order to kill herself. In this scenario, I would clearly have been an accomplice in her death, but she would equally clearly have been the one to take the final step.

Designating the killing of a patient as physician-assisted suicide is supposed to shift the responsibility from the physician to the patient. But it was obvious to me that Claire Renan wanted me to take a direct, active role in ending her life, a life that could readily have been maintained for a considerable period of time. Simply renaming the deed did nothing to lessen my sense of dismay, even dread, at the prospect of conspiring to bring Claire Renan's life to a premature end. I preferred to acknowledge explicitly that honoring the request of a patient to help in terminating life was euthanasia, albeit voluntary euthanasia.

Calling it euthanasia did not make it wrong any more than calling it physician-assisted suicide made it right. In fact, I was perfectly willing to accept that killing was not invariably wrong. Killing in self-defense and killing in the context of war, I thought, were morally justifiable.[18] And withholding or withdrawing medical treatment, with the knowledge that this would result in death from underlying disease, also seemed eminently justifiable.[19] But killing to end suffering did not seem consistent with a physician's role of curing and caring.

Claire Renan thought that using medicine to end her life was perfectly consistent with a physician's mission. From her point of view, it was in fact my obligation to end her suffering. If killing her was the only way I could eradicate the emotional pain she was experiencing, then it was my duty to kill her. She also felt that she had a right to live and die in accordance with her view of what constituted a good life. Who was I to insist that she live on when she was ready to go? Two of the cardinal tenets of contemporary medical ethics, the principles of patient autonomy or self-determination and of beneficence or acting in the patient's best interest, seemed to support Claire Renan's position. Did I feel uneasy merely because of fear of criminal liability? Was I distressed because I would be venturing into uncharted waters, engaging in a practice that the majority of Americans believe should be available to them but that most would not actually want to use,[20] a practice that was not sanctioned by either the courts or professional medical associations?

I tried very hard to understand why I was so reluctant to do Claire's bidding. I concluded that part of my distress stemmed from concern about what participating in euthanasia would do to me.[21] I worried about the "slippery slope" argument: once killing became acceptable in some circumstances, it would become legitimate in other situations as well. After all, if competent patients had the right to demand euthanasia, then surely incompetent patients could not be deprived of that right, which would open the door to involuntary euthanasia. This is in fact under consideration in Holland, where euthanasia is technically illegal, but where it is not prosecuted provided certain conditions are met.[22] The possibility of legitimizing the right of surrogates to choose death for their wards was frightening because it raised the specter of German physicians collaborating with their Nazi compatriots in the murder of "undesirables." It was also frightening because I could imagine that if I agreed to assist my patients in suicide, my personal moral sense would gradually be eroded: having tried physician-assisted suicide and found it painless, I might more easily be prevailed upon to assist in ending the lives of those who were a little less clear about their desires.

There was another reason why I rejected Claire Renan's plea to "do something" to help her, why I bristled at her accusations of abandonment. Underlying the argument that a physician was obligated to act in his patient's best interest and therefore had to kill if this provided relief of suffering was an unstated assumption: that a physician's role is to cure suffering. A physician's duty is undeniably to try to relieve suffering, but doctors can no more be expected to cure suffering than they can be expected to cure chronic diseases such as arthritis or diabetes.[23] Western physicians over the past decades have been accused of focusing on curing at the expense of caring.[24] When it came to pain, Claire shared the physicians' mystique and wanted cure, not palliation. She wanted a quick fix, total relief, and when she found that was impossible she preferred death to continued existence.

The pain and suffering that Claire wanted fixed were particularly difficult to treat because they were emotional, not physical. She really had very little physical pain, except when she was constipated and had to strain to move her bowels past the tumor in her rectum. Her pain arose from her loss of independence, from the shame of her incontinence, from fear of further decay and disintegration. The argument that physician-assisted suicide should never be necessary if modern pain control methods were correctly used simply did not apply to Claire Renan. There were no medications that could relieve her suffering. Antidepressants had not worked; anti-anxiety medications had not helped and had made her confused; attempts at psychotherapy were unsuccessful. But was I a failure as a doctor if I could not cure Claire Renan's psychic pain, her overwhelming sadness and rage over aging? My role was supportive. I could try to make Claire as functional as possible during her final months or years. This entailed such things as blood transfusions to improve her strength and prescribing a wheelchair to help her maintain some degree of mobility. I could try to make her as comfortable as possible by treating her arthritic pain with medication and trying to regulate her bowels with a judiciously selected combination of stool softeners and cathartics. I could provide relief by simply being there, by acknowledging her misery and promising not to abandon her. But I increasingly felt that suffering is part of the human condition. While I do not mean to suggest that suffering is good—that it builds character or is spiritually redeeming[25]—neither do I think that physicians must at all cost obliterate suffering, if necessary by causing death.

It would have been easier had Claire Renan been a religious

woman. Then, perhaps, she would have found meaning in suffering through her faith. As it was, the only meaning she could impute to her pain was that through her suffering she was linked to all of humankind; she was sharing a quintessentially human experience, analogous in its way to passion or ambition. I could try to help Claire see suffering in this light, I could ameliorate her pain, but I could no more cure her suffering than I could cure aging or stave off death.

Claire Renan was unusual in that she wanted to let go of life before her time had come, before she had developed irreversible, untreatable medical problems, even before she had any condition whose treatment was objectively burdensome. At the other end of the spectrum are patients—or, more often, families—who are unable to let go, who if given a choice are never able to decline a treatment that has some chance, however remote, of prolonging life.

Fortunately, most of the time patients, families, and physicians can come to an agreement about what constitutes a reasonable approach to care at the end of life. But there are clearly a number of obstacles to finding a sound approach to the care of the dying. It may not be clear beyond a reasonable doubt that a person is dying. The patient may, like Jennie Rosetti, be incapable because of illness of making decisions to limit care, leaving surrogates and the physician in the position of deciding what path to take. Or the patient may be perfectly lucid, like Claire Renan, but may make demands that the medical profession is not currently—and perhaps never should be—in a position to carry out. Occasionally it happens that it is quite clear that a person is dying, the individual is ready to accept the inevitability of an imminent demise, and the physician and other health care providers are able to work with the patient to ease the end of life.

The Hospice Approach

When Eleanor Richards first called me about her mother-in-law, I had no idea that I would soon be caring for a patient who was terminally ill. Eleanor Richards had called me because she was looking for a physician who would make house calls. The elder Mrs. Richards was housebound as a result of severe emphysema and arthritis. Because of her stiff, arthritic knees and the oxygen tank she used at all times, she was no longer able to climb down the stairs from her second-floor apartment to the front door. She had become a prisoner in her own home, leaving only when she summoned an ambulance because she could not breathe. Over the last several months, Carol Richards had been transported by ambulance to the local emergency room three times, where she was invariably admitted with the diagnosis of exacerbation of chronic obstructive lung disease.

Between hospitalizations, Mrs. Richards never saw her primary care physician. It was simply too much of an effort to get out of the house. In fact, only ambulance drivers were willing to carry her down the stairs on a stretcher, so even for routine medical appointments she needed an ambulance. The visiting nurse who checked on Mrs. Richards weekly urged her to have follow-up by a physician. Since her usual doctor did not make house calls, Mrs. Richards and her daughter-in-law decided to try a new doctor.

Because my practice was devoted exclusively to geriatric patients, some of whom are truly housebound, I tried to make home visits to a small number of patients who lived near the office. Carol Richards sounded like a very appropriate candidate for a house call.

Mrs. Richards lived in an old two-family house on a quiet residential street in a lower-middle-class suburb. A narrow, twisting staircase led to Mrs. Richards's apartment. Five rooms should have been ample for one 76-year-old woman, but they were cluttered with memorabilia and imposing furniture that seemed too large, as though it had previously occupied a stately Victorian home. The curtains were drawn, the lighting was poor, and the thermostat must have been set at 80 degrees. I was tempted to fling open the windows and let the cool fall air blow away the smell of yesterday's dinner. But this was Carol Richards's home, not my office, so I restrained myself and focused my attention on my new patient.

She was tiny: probably no more than four feet ten inches and 75 pounds. She had not always been quite so short: she had lost easily three inches from the osteoporosis-induced curvature of her spine. She looked younger than her 76 years, probably because her smooth black face was totally free of wrinkles. She walked with a walker, wheeling her portable oxygen tank behind her. She was short of breath just from walking the ten feet from her living room sofa to her bedroom, where I was to examine her. With difficulty, she climbed onto her bed and lay down. She was breathing rapidly and her pulse was racing from the exertion. Although she was not wheezing, there was very poor air flow into her lungs, indicating severe obstructive lung disease. Her lips were not blue, so she was getting a reasonable amount of oxygen. There was nothing to suggest heart failure, which often complicates severe emphysema. In fact, apart from her lung disease, Mrs. Richards's only other medical problem was her arthritis. She had no swelling of her joints, but her knees creaked when she bent them: it was the sound of bone rubbing against bone, with none of the cushioning normally provided by a well-lubricated joint.

I asked Mrs. Richards how she was getting along. She said she managed with difficulty to get out of bed in the morning and that she often just threw a housecoat over her nightgown. She made herself a cup of tea for breakfast. The morning was spent reading the newspaper, waiting for the daily call from her son, and waiting for the mail. At 11:30, she received a warm home-delivered meal from the meals-on-wheels program. She chatted with the man who brought the food about the weather and the day's menu. After lunch Mrs. Richards typically took a nap. Twice a week a home health aide came to give her a sponge bath. Once a week a homemaker did some shopping for her, vacuumed the apartment, and did a load of laundry. The rest of the day Mrs. Richards watched television. She had formerly spent a great deal of time crocheting, and she proudly showed me some of her handiwork. For over a year she had been unable to crochet because the arthritis in her hands interfered with her fine motor coordination.

For dinner she heated up leftovers or made herself a can of soup.

The evenings were long and lonely, so especially in winter when it got dark early, Mrs. Richards went to bed at eight. On weekends there were no meals-on-wheels, and her daughter-in-law and grandchildren took turns coming over for a visit and bringing a hot lunch. She had no brothers or sisters in the area: she had moved to Massachusetts from South Carolina as a young woman seeking her fortune, and what family remained still lived in the South. Most of her friends had either died or moved away. She was lucky, however, that she had made a community for herself in the local Baptist church. She had been a member of the choir in the past when she could sing without getting short of breath, and had been involved in church picnics and bazaars, in staffing soup kitchens, and in teaching in Sunday school. Once she became homebound, the minister came to visit her frequently, and members of the church dropped in weekly.

Mrs. Richards had a lifeline button that she wore around her neck with which to summon an ambulance if she became acutely ill and was unable to reach the telephone. A nurse came from the visiting nurses' association several times after each hospitalization to check on her respiratory status. Once she had been found to be medically stable, she was discharged from the VNA's case list. A technician from the company supplying her oxygen visited every so often to check the equipment. That was the sum total of the events in Carol Richards's life.

We talked for a while about her view of her life. Yes, she was lonely. No, she did not feel depressed. She wished she could get out of the house, but she had no desire to move to a first-floor apartment. She really could not have a pet to keep her company because she could barely take care of herself and was not about to start worrying about cleaning cages or putting out kitty litter. Obviously she could not walk a dog. What she missed above all else was a cigarette.

Over the course of the next few months, I got to know Carol Richards better, both her medical problems and her philosophy of life. It was after another stay in the hospital that we had a long talk about her wishes for future medical care. She had been admitted, as usual, for shortness of breath, precipitated this time by an upper respiratory infection. The oxygen level in her blood when she had arrived in the emergency room was a record low for her—30; it usually hovered in the 50s on room air and would have been in the 90s in a healthy person. The partial pressure of carbon dioxide in her blood, which would measure around 40 in a person with normal lungs and was usually 50 to 60 in Mrs. Richards, had climbed all the way to 80. No matter how hard and fast she breathed, she was unable to expel more carbon dioxide and to inhale more oxygen through her lungs and into her circulation. She was given a mask with 100 percent oxygen; she also got intravenous fluids because she was slightly dehydrated, antibiotics because her sputum showed evidence of a possible bacterial infection, and chest physical therapy to help her cough up the thick secretions that were blocking her bronchial tubes. Both the pulmonary specialist and I thought it near-miraculous that Mrs. Richards had survived without being put on a respirator, a machine to breathe for her.

During my first home visit after she had returned from the hospital, I asked how it had felt to be so desperately air-hungry. It was truly awful, Mrs. Richards told me. But then, without my even asking, she volunteered that she would not under any circumstances wish to be put on a respirator. She had said so before, and her son and daughter-in-law knew that was how she felt, and she had not changed her mind. She had discussed her situation with her minister, and he understood that her time would come soon. Mrs. Richards knew that her lungs were so severely damaged that she was in effect dying of emphysema. If she reached the point at which she could only be kept alive by a ventilator, it would in all likelihood mean that her lungs had deteriorated to such an extent that she would never be able to breathe without a machine. And she felt that life in a hospital bed, tethered to a large and noisy machine, unable to speak because of the tube inserted in her trachea, was no life at all.

I decided to push her a bit. Was her present life satisfactory? Not great, but a life. Was it worth living? Yes; she had no interest in terminating her current life. Three years ago, or five years ago, if she had been told she would be homebound, dependent on oxygen, a virtual recluse, would she have thought that was a life worth living? She wasn't sure. Might life on a ventilator similarly seem to be unendurable, a nightmare, whereas in fact if it came to that she would put up with it as she had with so much? Mrs. Richards thought for a long time. No, she finally said, this was different. She understood that now she was slowly dying. When she could no longer breathe for herself, she would be dead. There was no point pretending it wasn't so and putting her on a machine to prolong her dying.

One month later, Carol Richards was again hospitalized. This time, after a week of the now-customary routine, she remained short of breath even when sitting in a chair. The hospital staff caring for her did not see how she could possibly go home in her condition. They felt she should be in a chronic care hospital or a nursing home, where she would have around-the-clock medical attention. Mrs. Richards disagreed. She had no desire to spend her remaining days in an institution, any more than she wished to finish her life on a ventilator. She felt she could still cope at home: she would just move more slowly and be a little more uncomfortable. There was not really very much that a nurse or a doctor could do for her, she felt, though it would be nice to have someone with her if she became extremely short of breath. She also acknowledged that whenever her breathing deteriorated markedly, when the oxygen level plummeted and the carbon dioxide soared, she became slightly confused. And when she was confused, she was not safe by herself.

We agreed that if Mrs. Richards was to go home, she would need a good deal more in the way of home services. We also agreed that the goal of medical care at this stage of her illness was to maintain comfort. I suggested that Mrs. Richards might benefit from becoming a hospice patient.

She was rather taken aback. She had heard of hospice in connection with cancer patients, and did not see how hospice, whatever that was, could apply to her. For a moment she thought I had mixed her up with another patient and that I believed she had lung cancer. Then she thought that perhaps she did have lung cancer, and everyone had been keeping the truth from her. I reassured her that to the best of my knowledge she did not have lung cancer, but hastened to add that her emphysema was every bit as lethal as cancer. In some respects it was more lethal, since many forms of cancer are treatable and some are curable, whereas the damage done to Mrs. Richards's lungs was permanent and irreversible. Hospice, I explained, was a program for which anyone with a terminal illness and a prognosis of six months or less was eligible. She was skeptical: she had heard of inpatient hospice programs, and remained opposed to institutionalization in any kind of facility. She certainly did not want to move in with a group of dying strangers.

The hospice program I had in mind was home hospice. Mrs. Richards would remain in her home, and I would continue as her physician. But instead of receiving home care services from a variety of agencies, all her care would be coordinated by the hospice. Nurses specially trained in the care of terminally ill patients and dedicated to making the last months of life as comfortable as possible would see her—and would continue to visit even if she temporarily was medically stable. If the shortness of breath became severe, the nurses had the technological know-how to administer morphine through a needle under the skin so Mrs. Richards would not feel as though she were suffocating. The hospice nursing staff was on call twenty-four hours a day for emergencies. They were prepared to do their best to ensure that their patients experienced a peaceful death and did not die alone. Associated with the hospice program were other professionals such as social workers, who also possessed expertise in death and dying.

It sounded like a good deal to Carol Richards. The only potential stumbling block was that the hospice director required that a friend or family member be available to provide emotional support and to make a commitment to a certain amount of hands-on caregiving. Mrs. Richards's only child, Paul, was a traveling salesman who was out of town a good part of the time. He seemed to be comfortable with the idea of his mother receiving palliative care and accepted that she was not going to be around much longer. But he was squeamish about the prospect of actually having to touch his mother, to help bathe her or dress her or clean her up if she did not quite make it to the bathroom in time. Her church family, while extremely supportive, could not be asked to take on such a major commitment. That left Eleanor, Carol Richards's daughter-in-law, as the obvious candidate for the position of chief caretaker. Eleanor had always selflessly made herself available to her three children. Now that her youngest had finally left home at age 28, she found herself called upon to help care for an ailing mother-in-law.

Carol Richards did not want to burden her daughter-in-law, and I certainly did not want to pressure the daughter-in-law into accepting greater responsibility than she felt she could handle. I prevailed upon the family to meet with the hospice nurse to find out exactly what was involved. The nurse proved to be a good mediator as well as an outstanding salesperson. She saw that Mrs. Richards was very eager to enroll in the hospice program, which she regarded as her only alternative to a nursing home. She also recognized that Carol Richards would feel tremendously guilty if she made any further demands on her family. The nurse ingeniously argued that for the hospice plan to work, Mrs. Richards needed to pay for a few hours of private care a day to supplement what hospice and her daughter-in-law could reasonably be expected to provide. This simple proposal lightened the load for everybody just enough to make their responsibilities tolerable. Carol Richards was accepted into the hospice program.

Events moved quickly from that point. Two weeks later, Mrs. Richards's breathing worsened for no discernible reason. Maybe the colder weather had something to do with it. This time her heart began to fail, overburdened by the strain of pumping against the high blood pressure that had developed in her lungs as a complication of emphysema. Fluid backed up into Mrs. Richards's legs and began accumulating in her abdomen. I prescribed intravenous diuretics, which the hospice nurse administered at home. Gradually the fluid resolved, but Mrs. Richards was left even weaker than before. She stayed in her bedroom all the time, finding even the trip from her bed to her armchair or to the bathroom a strain.

Eleanor came each evening to help her mother-in-law back to bed, first making sure she had washed up and gone to the bathroom. The two women got into the habit of chatting for a while before Eleanor left. Perhaps because Mrs. Richards's mind was a little fuzzy from the chronically low oxygen, perhaps because of the intimacy into which they had been forced, she felt uninhibited in a way she had not experienced before. She talked about her son Paul as a child, recalling anecdotes from his high school days; she told about her work as a secretary during World War II. And Eleanor reciprocated, sharing her misgivings about how her grandchildren were being raised and her anxiety about the mental health of her oldest daughter.

Then Mrs. Richards caught a cold, and her breathing got even worse. She became too weak to get out of bed and began using a bedpan instead of the commode. What little she ate and drank had to be brought to her in bed. The hospice nurse felt she could no longer be left alone, and a personal care attendant was hired to be with her twelve hours a day. Eleanor decided she would stay overnight.

Eleanor could do this because she knew it would not last very long. By the second night, her mother-in-law was getting morphine. She had become so confused, agitated, and short of breath that we all felt it was time for gentle sedation. Mrs. Richards fell asleep with the morphine running into her and never woke up. Her breathing became shallower and shallower, and on the third night that Eleanor was with her, she stopped breathing altogether. Eleanor had dozed off, physically exhausted and emotionally drained, and woke up because the room suddenly seemed silent. She had never seen a dead person before and did not fully trust her diagnosis. She called the hospice nurse on duty, who came at once—at once being five in the morning—pronounced Mrs. Richards dead, and then sat with Eleanor for nearly an hour, talking about what she had just been through.

Perhaps the greatest testimonial to the virtues of hospice is the obituary I saw in the local paper after Carol Richards's death. In lieu of flowers, mourners were requested to send donations to the hospice program. I ran into Eleanor in the doctors' office building where I worked a few months later, by chance, when she was coming in for a routine visit herself. I mentioned the obituary, and Eleanor proceeded to tell me just how wonderful the hospice program had been for the entire family.

For Carol Richards, hospice had made it possible to die at home rather than in a hospital or a nursing home, which had been personally very important to her. It had been so important that she had been willing to stay at home even if it meant risking lying on the floor after a fall, unable to get up, or being alone and helpless when she became acutely short of breath. With the system of caretakers set up by the hospice and the ready availability of nurses, Mrs. Richards had not only been able to stay at home, but she had been as safe as she would have been in a nursing home. The hospice nurses had shown Eleanor and Paul how to help Mrs. Richards just enough so they would neither feel burdened by their participation in her care nor guilty about lack of involvement. When they were away from her, they had felt relaxed, confident that she was being well taken care of, and above all, reassured by the knowledge that she was not alone.

The involvement of hospice had not stopped with Carol Richards's death. Her primary nurse, Sherry, came to the funeral. June, the social worker who had met with Mrs. Richards on several occasions, paid a call to Paul and Eleanor a month later to see how they were doing. She recognized that the first few weeks after Mrs.

Richards's death would be so taken up with funeral arrangements, closing the apartment, paying outstanding bills, and other busy work that the family would be distracted from the pain of their loss. Once the visitors and the condolence cards stopped coming, Paul and Eleanor were expected to act as though everything were back to normal. They did not, however, feel ready to resume their previous routine. When June telephoned and asked if she could stop by, they felt she was like an emissary sent from heaven to give them news about Mrs. Richards. With June they did not have to keep a stiff upper lip and pretend that nothing momentous had happened: Eleanor could reveal how frightened she had been about being alone with someone who was dying; Paul could joke about what a wonderful device a urinal was and how it was too bad that women were not built to be able to use one; they could both cry.

Hospice care made sense to Carol Richards because she was convinced that her death was imminent and therefore felt that the goal of medical care was to ease her death rather than to fight for her life. On the basis of the information I had given her about her pulmonary functions and the oxygen levels in her blood and their prognostic significance, she realized that her death was inevitable no matter what medical interventions were undertaken—unless she chose to spend the rest of her days hospitalized, on a respirator. My estimate of her likelihood of making it through another winter without artificial respiration could, of course, have been wrong. More precisely, since I never said she had no chance of survival, she could have been one of the 10 or 20 percent of people who did pull through. Predictions by their very nature are probabilistic. I had not told Carol Richards with certainty that she would die within the next six months, but rather that her odds of survival were in the range of 10 to 20 percent. For some people, that would have been sufficient grounds for putting up with further hospitalizations, painful blood tests in which a needle would be inserted directly into an artery to measure oxygen and carbon dioxide levels, and the risk of infections, falls, and disorientation entailed by the hospital environment.[26] For Carol Richards, the indignities of repeated hospital care would have been worth enduring if she had had a 50 percent chance or greater of returning to her baseline state. For a 10 percent chance, or at most 20 percent, she was unwilling to take the gamble.

Enrolling in a hospice program did not mean forgoing all potential benefits of medical technology. Cecily Saunders, the British founder of the modern hospice movement, was not a Luddite, bent on destroying all vestiges of technology.[27] Resigning herself to dying did not mean that Carol Richards rejected medical care. Instead, it meant embracing a kind of care that harnessed medical science in the service of maintaining comfort. Mrs. Richards continued to use her home oxygen tank. When she filled up with fluid and oral diuretics proved useless, she permitted the nurses to administer intravenous diuretics. But in addition to conventional medical treatment for disease, she took advantage of special techniques for the control of pain and agitation. The hospice nurses were adept with a special pump that delivers a constant flow of morphine through a needle lodged under the skin. More traditional systems require an intravenous needle, which often comes out of the vein, resulting in pain and swelling at the point of entry. (Another approach—using a special patch impregnated with narcotics in a medium designed to permeate gradually into the underlying skin—was not available at the time of Carol Richards's terminal illness.) Mrs. Richards suffered from constipation in her final days, a frequent problem in immobile patients who eat little, drink less, and take constipating narcotics. Sherry, like most hospice nurses, had developed a level of sophistication about stool softeners, laxatives, and cathartics which clearly exceeded mine and that of most primary care physicians, for whom constipation is a minor and mundane problem.[28]

Hospice, as currently designed, is not for everyone. Not only must patients be ready to acknowledge that they are dying; they must also meet certain criteria specified by the government. Hospice is a Medicare benefit, for which Medicare patients are eligible if they are terminally ill with a life expectancy of six months or less, are unable to benefit from further curative therapy, are able to receive 80 percent of their care at home, and have a caregiver who will assume the responsibility for custodial care.[29] Fortunately, Carol Richards fit the increasingly stringent criteria. Other patients who fail to qualify, sometimes on a technicality, are not so lucky.[30] For Mrs. Richards, as for the majority of hospice patients who report a higher level of satisfaction with their care than conventional care patients,[31] it was a perfect match.

Hospice care could serve many more people than it currently does. The terminal nature of many kinds of cancer, particularly metastatic cancer, is widely accepted. From a statistical viewpoint, many other diseases share at least as gloomy a prognosis: cirrhosis of the liver, cardiomyopathy (a degenerative condition of the heart in which the pump function is severely impaired), and emphysema are a few examples of progressive disorders that bring their victims closer and closer to death. At some point—and this point needs to be identified clinically by physicians and accepted emotionally by the person suffering from the disease—medical therapy can no longer prolong life. Medical care can continue to be supportive and palliative, promoting comfort and maximizing quality of life for whatever time remains. This is precisely the kind of care in which hospice excels.

Everyone dies of something, and everyone dies eventually. The leading cause of death in the elderly is cardiovascular disease, with malignancy in second position, stroke in third, and chronic lung disease in fourth.[32] For some, the terminal event is a devastating illness that strikes seemingly randomly and unexpectedly, such as Jennie Rosetti's pneumonia. For many, the stroke or heart attack or bout of congestive heart failure is one of a long series of debilitating events, each of which reduces the individual to a lower level of functioning. All those people who are gradually declining, slowly but surely failing, ultimately cross the threshold into the realm of the dying. The challenge for medicine is to establish with greater accuracy when this occurs, and to teach patients that hospice-style care is the most conducive to their well-being once they have crossed the line.

❖ 4 ❖

Living with Limited Reserves:
The Frail Elderly

Tales of old people who are dying but are not allowed to die figure prominently in contemporary writing; the boundless energy and exciting exploits of the robust elderly are flashed before us in glowing popular accounts of the possibilities of old age; and the tragic plight of the demented is increasingly the subject of media attention, though often in the context of a scientific breakthrough that holds up the promise of a cure for Alzheimer's disease.[1] The unsung heroes of the elderly generation are those who are neither robust nor dying, and who are not necessarily mentally in decline, but rather who are physically frail.

Frail older people typically have no one overriding health problem. Instead they suffer from impairments in multiple domains, modest deficiencies in the function of their kidneys, heart, lungs, brain, and glands that collectively render them vulnerable to the slightest perturbation. They may become desperately ill with a simple case of the flu; they tend to become disoriented outside their neighborhood; they readily become dehydrated in the heat. The frail elderly simply have no physiological reserves on which to draw. They can function day-to-day, though sometimes only with considerable help from others, but they can be tipped over from a state of tolerable functioning to helplessness and illness with minimal provocation.

Addressing the medical problems of the frail is the bread and butter of geriatric medicine, but there is little poetry inspired by frailty. Autobiographical and fictional accounts of aging focus on the drama, but seldom on the prosaic details that make all the difference to the frail older person. I have yet to read a story in which the elderly protagonist describes his intense embarrassment upon suddenly developing incontinence, only to be rescued by a geriatric consultant who determines that his problem has been caused by the new blood pressure medication he is taking. The frail elderly are also sequestered from public view because they are often homebound or secluded in nursing homes. Despite their relative invisibility, 22 percent of women and 15 percent of men age 65 and over are regarded as frail, and the degree of disability rises markedly with age.[2] Medical decision making in this group is difficult precisely because when the frail get sick, they tolerate interventions poorly. The goal of treatment is usually the maintenance or restoration of functioning. But given the difficulty of treating without causing a cascade of unwanted complications, are there situations in which it makes sense to forgo what appears, technically, to be the best treatment? For individuals in whom the environment has a profound influence on both their emotional and physical coping abilities, are factors such as where and with whom they live as or more important than what medical treatment alternative they select? And finally, are there situations in which function has declined to such an extent that only palliative treatment is warranted, as with the dying elderly?

The perils of conventional, state-of-the-art medical care in the frail elderly are rarely taught to medical students. They are seldom discussed by physicians with patients or their families when talking about alternative approaches to treatment, or in obtaining informed consent for a surgical procedure. By the time I became involved in the care of Sam Schaeffer, this quintessentially geriatric perspective was too late to help.

One Complication after Another

Samuel Schaeffer was an 83-year-old man who could not be said to be vigorous or in very good health, but who was neither demented nor dying. He had a long list of medical problems, including diabetes, high blood pressure, congestive heart failure, psoriasis, and emphysema. He took at least one prescription medication for each of his illnesses, and some of the medications he took several times a day. Despite all attempts to simplify Mr. Schaeffer's medication regimen, he took nine pills on the best of days, and on the worst, when he developed bronchitis and a concomitant exacerbation of his breathing troubles, he took closer to fifteen pills. He checked his urine to see if his diabetes was under reasonably good control; he checked his own blood pressure to ensure that it was not excessively high; he weighed himself daily to be certain he was not filling up with fluid; and he took his own pulse to be sure it was neither too fast nor too slow. His physician had suggested substituting a blood test for the urine test to follow the status of his diabetes more precisely, but he balked at the prospect of pricking his own finger to measure his blood sugar.

Mr. Schaeffer liked to take a short nap in the afternoon, so he calculated that between his nap, the medications, and his own self-monitoring, he had about twelve productive hours a day. Those hours were good ones. He avidly read the newspaper, and he participated in a weekly discussion group of retired men that focused on political events. He was working on a memoir about life in New York City in the thirties and forties, where he had lived as a young man. Mr. Schaeffer spent several afternoons a week with each of two sets of grandchildren and, when he was up to it, watched them by himself for a few hours.

The summer after his eighty-third birthday, Mr. Schaeffer noticed that he was becoming increasingly fatigued. He found himself getting up at nine o'clock instead of his usual seven. He rarely managed to get out in the morning because it took him so long to get washed and dressed. Just performing his household chores—and his house was a compact four-room apartment—left him exhausted. He did not feel up to preparing much in the way of lunch, and despite a strong cup of coffee with whatever lunch he managed to throw together, he invariably dozed off afterward. His afternoon rest seemed to stretch from a 45-minute catnap to a two-hour siesta, following which he felt energetic enough to go out shopping or visiting or simply strolling. Though he became quite animated when he was with his family, even the company of his favorite daughter could not prevent him from being ready for bed by nine in the evening.

At first, his physician thought Mr. Schaeffer was depressed. He was lonely, having lost his wife a year earlier and having outlived many of his closest friends. He did not have any other signs of depression, however: he was not sad, his appetite was good, and there were plenty of things he was eager to do when he felt physically fit. A psychiatrist concurred: Mr. Schaeffer was a bit isolated, a bit lonely, but not clinically depressed. He was put through a battery of tests, searching for a cancer that might manifest itself only as chronic fatigue, but the tests were all negative. He had no anemia or metabolic problems such as an underactive thyroid gland. Test after test came back normal. Medications that might be causing or contributing to the fatigue were eliminated. Nothing helped.

Mr. Schaeffer gradually adjusted to his new, lower energy level. He no longer had the stamina to stay alone with his five-year-old grandchild, and he only attended his discussion group when he had a ride. He often fell asleep while reading the newspaper, but he still made it through the *New York Times* every day, he still visited with his family weekly, and he continued to work on his memoirs. He hired a homemaker to do his grocery shopping, his laundry, and to vacuum the apartment, and he had a hot meal delivered daily through the meals-on-wheels program.

At Thanksgiving, Mr. Schaeffer developed his first bout of pneumonia. It started with a cough and suddenly blossomed, producing disorientation and confusion. He was hospitalized and given oxygen and intravenous antibiotics; in a week he was home again, a bit weaker than his previous none-too-energetic self, but back to his usual activities.

Pneumonia came again in January. Then in March, when Mr. Schaeffer felt he had finally recovered from the pneumonia, he awoke in the night with crampy abdominal pain. He groped to the bathroom, clutching chairs and closet door handles along the way. He managed to lower himself onto the toilet seat just in time for the emergence of a copious amount of sticky black stool. He then proceeded to stand up and faint.

Mr. Schaeffer's one bit of good fortune was that he landed in a heap on his plush bath mat, avoiding striking his head on the hard tile floor or the porcelain fixtures. He rapidly regained consciousness, made it to the telephone to summon help, and was in the emergency room within an hour.

This time the problem was a bleeding duodenal ulcer, probably triggered by the medication he was taking for arthritis. Mr. Schaeffer's blood pressure was dangerously low, and he was profoundly anemic. After several blood transfusions, potent anti-ulcer medication, and discontinuation of the arthritis medication, he was remarkably improved. During the course of this hospitalization, a cardiologist evaluated him because of the chronic fatigue. The cardiologist ordered an echocardiogram, in which sound waves are bounced off the heart to delineate its function. To everyone's surprise, the echocardiogram revealed advanced aortic stenosis: a marked narrowing of the valve connecting the major ventricle of the heart to the aorta. Mr. Schaeffer had experienced several of the classic symptoms of aortic stenosis—shortness of breath from congestive heart failure and fainting. However, the congestive heart failure had been attributed to added stress on the heart from the pneumonia, and the fainting had clearly been related to the gastrointestinal bleeding. The third major symptom of aortic stenosis, chest pain, Mr. Schaeffer had never had.

The new diagnosis set off a round of consultations and discussions. Was the aortic stenosis severe enough to justify aortic valve replacement, a major surgical intervention? By the usual criteria, the narrowing was severe enough to warrant surgery. Was Mr. Schaeffer in good enough condition to tolerate cardiac surgery? The cardiologist did not think so. The cardiac surgeon asserted emphatically that Mr. Schaeffer was not a surgical candidate. He recommended instead a balloon valvuloplasty, a less invasive procedure in which a catheter is threaded through an artery into the heart and the thickened valve leaflets are compressed so as to allow greater blood flow through the valve. Mr. Schaeffer and his daughter Ruth decided to seek a second opinion.

They were introduced by a physician friend of Ruth's to another cardiac surgeon. This surgeon concurred that a valve replacement would be very risky in someone of Mr. Schaeffer's age and overall health status. On the other hand, he felt that with medical treatment alone, Mr. Schaeffer would develop more congestive heart failure, would probably have further episodes of syncope, and would most likely go on to develop chest pain. In addition, he felt the fatigue that had been plaguing Mr. Schaeffer for some time was almost undoubtedly due to diminished blood flow secondary to the narrowed valve. The surgeon felt that valvuloplasty was a vastly inferior procedure, with which the stenosis frequently recurred, and was only to be used if the patient absolutely would not or could not tolerate open heart surgery. Ruth concluded from the discussion that her father's only chance was to undergo surgery now, because later, when he was even more debilitated, there would likely be no one willing to operate.

I was called to see Sam Schaeffer in my role as a geriatrics consultant two days after the surgery. The surgeons had been able to take Mr. Schaeffer off the ventilator, removing the endotracheal tube from his throat and thus enabling him to speak for the first time since the operation. His daughter was thrilled that he had come through with flying colors and was eager to hear how he was feeling.

To her dismay, what he said made no sense whatsoever. He repeatedly insisted that he was in a delicatessen and was furious when he was not given a pastrami sandwich for lunch. He called the nurses waitresses and thought the surgical resident was the chef. Later on he seemed to understand he was in a hospital, but was adamant that he had to go to the bathroom to urinate even though he had a catheter in his bladder.

Nighttime was even worse. Mr. Schaeffer thought the respiratory therapist was attacking him when she began tapping on his chest to help clear the secretions from his lungs. He defended himself by taking a swing at her. He was convinced that the night nurse had stolen his watch. He heard the sirens of ambulances approaching the hospital, thought they were fire engines, and began screaming that he needed to get out because the building was on fire.

I regarded all this as fairly commonplace postoperative delirium. Elderly patients often become temporarily disoriented and confused when hospitalized, even those whose minds are normally reasonably intact. The intensive care unit itself, with its absence of days and nights, its incessant alarm bells and constant mechanical noises, has been known to produce "ICU psychosis." Both anesthesia and the medications frequently used in the postoperative period are well known to cause confusion in vulnerable elderly patients. Mr. Schaeffer had been under general anesthesia for six hours; he was now receiving morphine for pain; he was getting cimetidine, an anti-ulcer medication, to prevent a recurrence of his gastrointestinal bleeding; and a sedative had been prescribed to help him sleep at night—all of which can contribute to an acute confusional state.

I recommended that Mr. Schaeffer's morphine dose be reduced, that he be given antacids instead of cimetidine, and that the particular sleeping medication that had been selected be changed, since it frequently produces confusion in the elderly. Moreover, I suggested that Mr. Schaeffer be transferred out of the intensive care unit as soon as possible because the environment itself was detrimental to his recovery. The ICU nurses were all too glad to be rid of this agitated and belligerent patient, so Sam Schaeffer moved to a regular ward in record time.

Ruth was relieved to find her father mentally back to normal within another two days. This time, she was confident, he really had survived the surgery and would be fine. She was correct that he had survived the surgery; she was wrong about his being fine.

A day after arriving on the surgical floor, Mr. Schaeffer developed a fever. Low-grade postoperative fevers are common, but Mr. Schaeffer's temperature rose to 103 degrees. His white blood cell count, normally in the 6,000 to 8,000 range, rose to 20,000, strongly suggestive of an infection. He began to cough, and his lungs sounded congested. A chest X-ray confirmed that Mr. Schaeffer had another pneumonia. He had not been taking deep breaths because it hurt to breathe, his lower lungs had gradually collapsed, and he had become infected with the bacteria endemic in intensive care units.

This was not a simple pneumonia. Perhaps because the infecting organism was *Pseudomonas,* a particularly virulent bacterium, perhaps because he was already weakened from the recent surgery, Sam Schaeffer did poorly. Within a day he was back in the intensive care unit, intubated again.

With vigorous treatment and the vigilant care of the ICU nurses, he slowly improved. Once more, he was able to be weaned from the respirator. Once again, he was transferred upstairs. And once more his daughter told me smilingly that he was out of the woods. I was not so sure.

By this time, Mr. Schaeffer had been bedridden for two weeks. When he attempted to get out of bed, he discovered that he was far too weak to take even a single step on his own. I suggested that a physical therapist work with him to help him regain his strength. I also recommended that he be given a blood transfusion so that he would not tire with the slightest exertion. The cardiologist advised prescribing stronger diuretics to help remove fluid from his lungs.

Just as he was beginning to progress a little bit, he developed florid diarrhea.

The diarrhea was not, as Mr. Schaeffer first thought, a sign of gastrointestinal bleeding. Instead, it was a result of the antibiotics he had been receiving for his pneumonia: the antibiotics were conducive to the proliferation of another species of bacteria within the colon, bacteria which generated a toxin that in turn caused diarrhea. This *Clostridium difficile* colitis itself was treated with still other antibiotics. The colitis totally destroyed what appetite Mr. Schaeffer had. Between his lack of intake and his profuse output of liquid through his diarrhea, he became dehydrated. He went back on intravenous fluids; he lost five pounds; and instead of becoming stronger, he got weaker. The physical therapist had to put off working with him because he was too sick and too weak to be able to follow an exercise or walking program.

Suddenly Ruth became worried that her father would not be able to return to his apartment. She was beginning to see that he would be incapable of caring for himself for a long time. I suggested that she discuss with the hospital social worker the various alternatives— if he survived to be discharged. He might be eligible for a stay at a rehabilitation hospital, although he would only be a candidate for an inpatient rehabilitation program if he progressed under the tutelage of the physical therapist at the acute care hospital. Rehabilitation hospitals have their own admissions committees and make their own decisions about who is likely to benefit from their services, I explained. I could not guarantee that he would be accepted; the best I could do was to ensure that he was again evaluated and treated by the therapist and to document in the chart how well-motivated he was, how eager to regain his independence. If one rehabilitation hospital rejected Mr. Schaeffer—and I warned that such facilities are sometimes leery about accepting very elderly patients with multiple medical problems—the social worker could request that he be evaluated by another institution, perhaps one with a slightly less intensive program. All rehabilitation hospitals operate under federal reimbursement guidelines, I cautioned, which require that patients receive three hours of therapy a day,[3] so even the slowest-paced program is in fact quite intensive. The end result might be that Mr. Schaeffer would be refused admission by all the facilities consulted. If that happened, he might need to enter a nursing home.

Ruth was appalled. She could not conceive of her father in a nursing home. She was overwhelmed by the realization that surviving surgery had not meant her father would return to his baseline level of functioning. I pointed out matter-of-factly that many nursing home stays were short term, that a nursing home could serve as the ultimate "slow rehab" program. Once Mr. Schaeffer was ready to be discharged from the hospital, he could conceivably spend a few months at a nursing home recuperating and then go home.

Ruth was not the only one to be dispirited by the lengthy hospitalization. Mr. Schaeffer himself was extremely frustrated by his numerous setbacks. He had no recollection of the immediate postoperative period, but he recalled the pneumonia and was devastated by the colitis. Moreover, he did not take well to his invalid status. He constantly summoned his nurse for assistance. He complained to the dietician that the food was never warm enough. He complained to the man who collected the television rental fee that the price was exorbitant. He complained to his daughter that his roommate snored. Never an easy man to get along with, Mr. Schaeffer became distinctly ornery in the hospital.

I took the orneriness as a good sign. The fact that Mr. Schaeffer was well enough to eat food, to watch television, and to notice that he had a roommate was auspicious. I began to think that perhaps he would pull through.

Sam Schaeffer had been in the hospital for thirty-three days when he had a heart attack. He awoke in the early morning with crushing chest pain, unable to breathe. His newly repaired aortic valve was working fine, but one of the coronary arteries feeding the heart had become blocked. His ailing heart could not pump properly, which caused fluid to back up into his lungs. I remember him reaching out to me when I came to see him, crying, "Help, do something, I'm suffocating!" He was given oxygen, morphine, diuretics, and additional cardiac medications. He still could not catch his breath. For the third time during his hospitalization, he was intubated and brought to the intensive care unit. Several hours later, he had a cardiac arrest. Despite vigorous attempts to resuscitate him with chest compressions, electric shocks, and potent intravenous medications, Sam Schaeffer died.

His death does not prove that he should not have had the surgery. Some octogenarians do well with the operation. Suppose Sam had recovered and been able to return to his apartment. Suppose further that he had gone back home with renewed vitality, no longer chronically fatigued, that he had finished his memoirs and been able to take care of his grandchildren again. Would that prove that he should have had the surgery? Clearly, failure does not imply he should not have had the procedure any more than success indicates he should have had it. At issue, once again, is the fact of uncertainty in medicine.

Sam Schaeffer made a decision about his personal medical care on the basis of statistical evidence describing the experience of large numbers of people, none of whom was precisely like him. He, together with his daughter, needed to assess the risks and benefits of surgery and to evaluate the relative merits of an operation and of alternative treatment. He had a pretty good grasp of the alternatives: he could either continue with the status quo, with some minor adjustment in his medications to improve flow across the diseased heart valve, or he could undergo a valvuloplasty. The problem with valvuloplasties is that often the improvement is only temporary; within a year, close to 50 percent of patients have a recurrence of stenosis of their valve.[4]

What was not very well explained to the Schaeffer family was the nature of the risks entailed by the operation. The surgeon was explicit about the risks of dying: he emphasized that 15 percent of octogenarians undergoing open heart surgery die.[5] From Sam Schaeffer's point of view, this meant that 85 percent of patients survive. Moreover, he was not frightened of dying in the operating room. Although he very much wanted to live, the possibility of a quick, painless death under anesthesia was a risk he was willing to take in exchange for a good chance of a marked improvement in his quality of life. The cardiac surgeon also enumerated a series of less dramatic risks: significant blood loss necessitating transfusion, development of an irregular heartbeat, and so on. He did not fully communicate that one of the risks to Sam Schaeffer was something other than death or a single, isolated medical complication. Another risk was a series of complications, a relentless chain of problems, producing a prolonged period of disability and finally ensuing in death. The scenario that Sam and his daughter were totally unprepared for was precisely the one that he experienced: one setback after another, each disaster linked to the preceding one, each episode rendered more devastating by his growing weakness.

Unfortunately, such a cycle of illness begetting illness is far from uncommon in the frail elderly. That is just what it means to be frail. Frailty cannot be measured by the number of underlying diagnoses or by the number of medications; it certainly is not a function of age alone. The frail elderly are those who are likely to be tipped over by any physical stress, by anything that places additional demands on a system already operating at maximal capacity and without reserves. Mr. Schaeffer was someone whose organs worked well enough to keep him going under normal circumstances. His lungs were adequate for everyday activities, but after surgery he was too weak to take deep breaths and cough to clear his secretions. He therefore developed a small amount of collapse of the air sacs at the bases of his lungs, a common postoperative condition. When a slightly impaired immune system and dangerous ambient bacteria were thrown into the equation, the result was a severe pneumonia. Similarly, his bowels had worked satisfactorily at home, but when given antibiotics for treatment of his pneumonia, he developed colitis. The *Clostridium difficile* bacterium that produced the colitis may have been living peacefully in his intestines even before the hospitalization—or he may have acquired it after the surgery or during a prior hospital stay. But in the presence of antibiotics, the *Clostridium difficile*'s natural adversaries are killed off, allowing them to multiply uncontrollably and to produce disease. Mr. Schaeffer's brain had also been functioning well before he was admitted to the hospital. When exposed to narcotics, anesthetics, and the ICU environment, his brain was unable to adapt, and the results were disorientation, impaired attention, lethargy, and even hallucinations and paranoia.

If Sam Schaeffer had known that he had a significant chance not merely of death but of experiencing a nightmarish cascade of catastrophes, would he have opted for surgery? Would the considerably lesser risks of valvuloplasty have made that procedure more alluring, despite its high relapse rate? It is this kind of death that is feared by many who complete living wills rejecting "heroic" or "extraordinary" measures. And it is this kind of terrifying tailspin toward death that has led observers to accuse physicians of willfully tormenting their patients in order to be paid for more hospital visits.[6]

Physicians do not wish to torment their patients. They do have difficulty withholding therapy for seemingly reversible conditions, and thus have trouble halting the flow of treatments once the machinery of medicine is set in motion.[7] Perhaps if patients understood the risks of the roller coaster ride—along with the risks of dying or of isolated medical problems—when they made weighty medical decisions, fewer would embark upon the ride in the first place.

The major decision Sam Schaeffer was called upon to make about his health care involved choosing between treatment options: valvuloplasty versus surgery versus medical therapy. As he suffered setback after setback, he might have been asked to decide whether he would opt not to be resuscitated in the event that his heart stopped. If he had chosen a do-not-resuscitate status, then he would have been spared the ultimately fruitless attempts to revive him when his heart ceased beating. If he had lived longer, he might have found that where he lived was just as important to his quality of life as his medical care. His daughter was just beginning to realize that if he survived he would not be able to go back home, at least not initially, and certainly not without substantial outside help. For some frail elders, the environment in which they live is critical not only to their comfort and sense of well-being, but even to the management of their medical problems.

A New Kind of Therapy

As a geriatrician, I spend a good deal of my time figuring out how to keep my patients at home, out of a nursing home. I seek to optimize their functioning—to improve their gait, to stop any medications that might make them confused, to diagnose and treat incontinence. I also work with numerous community agencies to help establish a care plan—a network of household and personal services that facilitate their staying at home. Typically, when the plan does not work out or the patient is too compromised to remain at home, I feel that I have failed. In reality, admission to a nursing home is often a welcome relief for the patient, as well as for family members, who are often exhausted and burned out.

Grace Fitzgerald had been my patient for a long time. I had taken care of her husband, who had himself entered a nursing home when Grace could no longer take care of him. I had been at his bedside when he died, for which Grace was deeply grateful. A year after his death, Grace decided her house was too large for her—with four bedrooms and three stories, it was too much to keep up. She moved in with her daughter Sally, who had never married and who worked as an executive secretary in a downtown law office.

Sally fixed up a room for her mother and installed an adjoining bathroom for her. She cooked dinner for the two of them when she got home from work, and they enjoyed each other's company during the evening meal. Sally did the shopping and the heavy cleaning, leaving the dishes and the dusting for her mother. On weekdays, Sally was up and out of the apartment before Grace had even gotten up. In the evening, Grace usually was ready for bed by nine, so she only saw her daughter a few hours a day. On weekends Sally took her mother out to a movie or shopping for clothes, and they treated themselves to dinner out every Sunday. It was a comfortable, easy existence for Grace.

The days started to become a problem for Grace when her arthritis acted up, making it difficult for her to get up from a chair by herself. When she did manage to get up, her joints were so stiff and painful that it took her a good five minutes to reach the bathroom. I tried her on a variety of anti-inflammatory medications, with modest success. She was evaluated by a physical therapist at home, who ordered a special chair for her that virtually ejected her from the seat. The therapist also arranged for a variety of devices to be installed throughout the apartment: a raised toilet seat and grab bars at selected locations. She prescribed exercises and heat treatments for Grace, which resulted in some degree of improvement. I sent Grace to see a rheumatologist, who injected her knees with steroids, providing significant pain relief. The pain was under control, but Grace remained extremely slow. She coped, however, until she developed a flareup of her Crohn's disease.

Crohn's disease had been with Grace for thirty years. An inflammatory bowel disease, it flared periodically, producing diarrhea and crampy abdominal pain. Grace had had a relatively mild case: she had never required hospitalization for prolonged bowel rest during a relapse; she had never had fistulas or abscesses or other complications necessitating surgery; and she had been symptom-free for several years. Out of the blue, for no discernible reason, Grace began to develop bloody diarrhea. She had a low-grade fever, she was in pain, and she worried that she would not reach the bathroom in time.

I visited Grace at home and found her distraught. From a technical point of view, she was not so ill that she unequivocally had to be hospitalized. I thought it at least possible that she would recover from the exacerbation of the Crohn's disease with a course of steroids and a clear liquid diet. I suggested that I could arrange for a visiting nurse to check on her daily, and for a home health aide to spend an hour or two a day on personal care. Grace looked at me imploringly and burst into tears. Sally, who had stayed home from work to care for her mother and to be certain to be present for my visit, glared at me and said in no uncertain terms: "My mother is a sick woman. She needs to be in the hospital."

I got the message. Whatever the facts—and certainly a case could be made for intravenous fluids and for keeping Grace strictly n.p.o. (nothing by mouth)—there were compelling social reasons for hospitalization. Grace could not be left alone even for a minute, because she was terrified that she would soil herself from the diarrhea. Medicare would not pay for community service agencies to supply eight hours of care a day to Grace; Sally was unable to take off more time from work to care for her mother; and Grace did not have the financial resources to pay privately for extensive home care.

The upshot was that I admitted Grace to the hospital. She stayed for ten days, during which time she was evaluated by a gastroenterologist, given intravenous fluids and steroids, and transiently given high-dose antibiotics for a suspected intra-abdominal abscess which proved to be a false alarm. Ultimately, she was discharged home, exhausted because the noise and the bustle had prevented her from sleeping well, anemic from her illness and from the daily blood drawings, and terribly anxious that she would relapse.

I tried to reason with Grace, pointing out that her disease had always been quite mild and that it had been two years since her last attack. I even tried to joke with her, pointing out that she usually had flareups around her birthdays and that she would not have a birthday for another year. She was in no mood for joking. Grace was gripped by anxiety, overwhelmed by the fear of being alone, obsessed by the image of bloody diarrhea dripping down her recalcitrant legs onto her hopelessly inadequate knees. She had a history of anxiety, and had done well before with short-term treatment using tranquilizers. I prescribed low doses of the same medication she had used previously, gradually increasing the amount until she was able to get through the day without episodes of sweating, tremulousness, and sheer panic.

It seemed that matters were under control: I saw Grace for a follow-up visit in the office and she had neither diarrhea nor shakes. She was making do at home. She had decided that the Sunday evening restaurant excursions and the shopping trips were too much for her, so she almost never left the apartment. She was bored and had become irritable and demanding; she wanted her daughter to stay home all day on weekends to play Scrabble and bridge. Instead, Sally invested in a VCR and supplied her mother with a new movie to watch every few days. The VCR was the basis of an uneasy truce between the two women.

The cease-fire collapsed a few weeks later. I got a message from Sally that she was on her way to the hospital emergency room with her mother. Grace, it turned out, was not herself: she was confused and disoriented. She thought she was back in her old home and kept repeating that she needed to visit her husband (long dead) in the nursing home. One minute she was quite animated, and the next she was drifting off to sleep. When I came to see her in the emergency room, she thought I looked familiar, but could not quite place me. Once again she was hospitalized, this time to search for the cause of her precipitous change in mental status.

At first I thought Grace was having a complication of the Crohn's disease—perhaps an intestinal infection, since infections sometimes manifest themselves by causing confusion in the elderly. But there was no elevated white blood cell count or fever to suggest infection, no abnormalities on X-ray, no bacteria in the bloodstream. Metabolic studies were normal too, including calcium and thyroid tests. I was perplexed, as were the other physicians caring for Grace.

Two days later, Grace was noted to have a rapid pulse and elevated blood pressure. At the same time, we received the results of the toxic screen that had been ordered on admission. The amount of benzodiazepine in her blood was markedly elevated for an 80-year-old woman. The pieces of the puzzle began to fit together: Grace Fitzgerald had become delirious from overmedicating herself with sedatives, and now she was jittery from withdrawal. Moreover, the irritability I had observed a few weeks earlier had probably been a sign of growing tranquilizer-dependence. Grace remained in the hospital for a week as she was gradually weaned from the offending medication. She was seen by a psychiatrist and put on a medication for panic attacks, one with less potential for abuse—a monoamine oxidase (MAO) inhibitor.

A week after Grace returned from the second hospitalization, I got a call from Sally. What would the problem be this time, I wondered? Could Grace have eaten one of the foods that was strictly forbidden to people taking an MAO inhibitor, and thus precipitated a hypertensive crisis? Was it her arthritis? Or the Crohn's again? Sally sounded very tired. It was no emergency, she told me. Her mother was doing as well as could be expected. It was she, Sally, who was having a problem. Her mother's hospitalization had provided a needed break for her, and now that her mother was back, she was again overwhelmed. Grace called her at least twice a day at the office. She complained about her daughter's cooking, maintaining that the diarrhea would come back if she didn't have her food cooked just so. Grace got up every night to go to the bathroom and had begun waking up her daughter to help her get out of bed. Sally felt she could not go out in the evening or on the weekends unless she found a companion to stay with Grace—and Grace protested that none of the sitters were satisfactory. Sally had started dating a co-worker from her office during her mother's hospitalization, and she was afraid that the relationship would go nowhere—like all her previous romantic entanglements—because of her mother's dependence on her. Sally started to cry on the telephone. Between the sobs, I heard her whisper: "I'm starting to hate my mother."

I suggested adult day care—a program to provide socialization and a modicum of nursing care to homebound elderly people—but we quickly realized that would not solve the problem. Day care ran from eight-thirty to two o'clock. It would break up the monotony of the long days, and it would give Sally a few hours when she could be safe from anxious phone calls and free of fear that some catastrophe would befall her mother in her absence. But it would do nothing about the evenings, the nights, and the endless weekends. Moreover, day care would create new problems. Grace would have to be dressed and ready to leave the apartment by eight o'clock. Normally she did not even get up before nine. Her entire routine would be disrupted if she were to try to be ready for the van at eight in the morning—and Sally would undoubtedly be called upon to help her wash, dress, and eat breakfast in time.

Respite care was another solution, albeit a temporary one. As a provider of care to her elderly mother, Sally was eligible for a certain number of hours of respite care a year—essentially babysitting services to give Sally some time off from her otherwise endless responsibilities. We concluded that the best solution was to hire private caretakers for Grace, as we had discussed when her Crohn's disease flared. Sally calculated that her mother would need help twelve hours a day—which would still leave Sally the night shift seven days a week. A live-in companion, which would have been cheaper since meals and lodging would be provided, was out of the question because the Fitzgeralds did not have sufficient space in their apartment. Twelve hours of help would cost $120 a day. Even if Sally took care of her mother on weekends in addition to handling the nights, Grace would use up her savings in four months.

Finding a qualified and compatible caretaker was not trivial either. In fact, Sally ended up with a patchwork arrangement involving three different women in order to get sixty hours a week of help. Together with Grace, she decided on a schedule of ten hours a day during the week and five hours on Saturday and Sunday, so Sally would have a little time for herself. It took running an ad in the paper, screening thirty individuals on the telephone, and interviewing ten people before Sally found women who she thought would work out.

The first week was rocky. Grace complained so bitterly about the way one of her aides did the housework that the aide quit. A second aide decided she would prefer taking care of an infant to dealing, as she put it, with a demanding old lady, so she gave notice. Sally had to take several days off from work to help her mother and to start all over with the search for aides. This time she contacted certified home health agencies, even though the rates were higher, in the hope that the caretakers would prove more reliable. At the very least, she hoped, the agency would supply backup personnel if the usual provider was out sick or quit.

The second week went considerably more smoothly. Grace began to develop a good relationship with one of her trio of assistants— Ann, a warm, hard-working woman from Barbados who was the first person Sally had hired. Ann had four young children, so she came at 8:30 in the morning, after she had gotten her children off to school. She left at 2:30 so as to be able to pick her children up from school. Ann helped Grace wash up in the morning, and served her both breakfast and lunch. She did a load of laundry, washed the dishes (sometimes including a sinkful from the previous evening), did another hour's worth of household chores, and spent the remaining time talking to Grace, listening to talk shows with her, and going on short, slow walks together.

Grace thrived with Ann's attention. Ann did not get angry or upset when Grace had a panic attack; she was calm and unflappable. Her cooking featured Caribbean island recipes, which she said would calm Grace's anxiety. Grace dutifully gobbled down the spicy foods which she would previously have avoided. Her anxiety attacks became less frequent, whether because of the food or the cook. After Ann went home, either Susie or Pat came, depending on the day of the week. Grace complained that Susie spent too much time watching the soaps and that the apartment needed a good cleaning each time Pat vacuumed. She did not think they were worth their wages, but grudgingly acknowledged that she needed them. Just how desperately Grace depended on her assistants became painfully evident shortly after the routine appeared to be firmly established.

It was a Monday afternoon, and Ann had just left to pick up her children from school. Pat, the afternoon aide, was due any minute. Grace was sitting in her recliner, reading a book. Every time she heard a car stop outside the building, she looked up at the door, expectantly. She glanced repeatedly at her watch. At three o'clock, she telephoned Pat's home. There was no answer. At 3:15, she called her daughter, who was in a meeting and unable to come to the phone. At 3:30, she broke into a cold sweat. Her heart began pounding. She began to feel that she could not breathe. Just when she was convinced that she was about to suffocate to death, what she had always dreaded happened: she felt an overwhelming urge to defecate, she stood up, and a flood of liquid stool gushed down her legs. Grace stood in the middle of the living room floor, effectively paralyzed. Gradually, the tight feeling in her chest subsided and her heart slowed from a gallop to a trot. She brushed the beads of sweat from her forehead and pushed the damp curls out of her face. She began walking, ever so slowly, to the bathroom, leaving a trail of stool behind her. Mustering all her resources, Grace managed to remove her soiled clothes. She made her way to her clothes closet and found a clean bathrobe. But bending down to wash her legs was beyond her. Stepping over the side of the tub to take a shower was totally out of the question. She suddenly realized that she could not escape from the foul odor that overwhelmed her, since she was at its epicenter. There was nothing to do but cry.

An hour later, Sally Fitzgerald's meeting was over and she got the message to call her mother. Within minutes, she was at the apartment bathing Grace, washing out the soiled clothes, and frantically calling Pat. When Pat finally answered the telephone later that evening, she announced that she was very sorry, but she had had severe cramps that day and had not felt like coming. Sally fired her on the spot.

Grace, who by this time had pulled herself together remarkably well, sat down with her daughter over a cup of tea. It was really very simple, she observed. She had to enter a nursing home. She had one wonderful caregiver—Ann—but the others were unreliable, and there was no guarantee they could find more responsible ones. It was awful for Grace and intolerable to Sally to depend on a few individuals for Grace's safety and Sally's peace of mind. In any event, the money would run out soon.

Sally was devastated, but she had to agree. She took the rest of the week off to visit nursing homes. Ann would stay on until a place was found, with Sally taking over after she left in the afternoon. There was a tremendous amount to do: Grace needed to be assessed by a government agency to determine her appropriateness for a nursing home and her "level of care"; a Medicaid application had to be filled out so that Medicaid would kick in once Grace's dwindling savings were depleted. And above all, the Fitzgeralds needed to find a nursing home that was clean, provided quality care, and was not unreasonably far away.

Fortunately, the director of the nursing home where Grace's husband had lived—and died—remembered the Fitzgeralds. Through a combination of luck and compassion, Grace had a room at the Silver Days Nursing Home a mere two weeks from the infamous day on which Pat failed to show up.

As it happened, Silver Days was one of the nursing homes I visited, so I was able to keep Grace as a patient. When I saw her a day after her arrival for the obligatory post-admission physical examination, she was downcast. She missed the apartment; she missed her daughter; she missed Ann. She could no longer decide when to have her meals or whether she wanted a bath. The nursing home had a schedule, and she had to adhere to it. She had a roommate— a sweet old lady who was stone deaf and had coughing spells in the middle of the night. Grace had not had a roommate since graduating from college sixty-five years earlier—unless she counted her husband. But she had chosen her husband. The roommate, while pleasant enough, was someone with whom she had next to nothing in common.

By the time of my next visit, thirty days later, Grace had arranged for her recliner to be brought from home—the special chair that helped eject her from the seat so she could get up on her own. It had been shampooed after the accident. It filled up a significant fraction of the space in her room, but it afforded her a welcome sense of freedom. In addition, Grace was able to arrange to have a telephone installed in her room. She did not abuse it—she rarely called Sally at work—but it permitted her to remain in contact with her few friends, her daughter, and Ann, with whom she spoke regularly.

Over the next year, Grace Fitzgerald had no further panic attacks and no flareups of her Crohn's disease. Her joints functioned well enough to permit her to ambulate with a walker throughout the nursing home and to go on all the outings arranged by her daughter or by the home. Sally kept her job, went through a series of romantic attachments, and finally moved in with another woman her own age.

For Grace Fitzgerald, it was just as important where she received her medical care as which tests, drugs, and other treatments she had. Her medication regimen was identical at home and in the nursing home, yet once in the nursing home she not only ceased to have flareups of Crohn's disease or anxiety attacks, but her arthritis, which had become increasingly debilitating, suddenly became tolerable. The aides in the nursing home found they did not have to do much for Grace: she could dress herself, she could eat unassisted, she could walk to the dining room alone, she could even get out of a chair without help once she had her special ejector seat. All they did on a routine basis was to give her a shower. What the nursing home provided for Grace was security, the certainty of the availability of around-the-clock help if she needed it. It also supplied her with three meals a day, fresh linen, and laundry service, all without her having to go shopping or hire homemakers. And finally, despite the disdain she felt for her hearing-impaired room-mate, Grace thrived on the companionship she found in the nursing home. She quickly established a good relationship with the head nurse on the day shift on her floor. She found she could confide in the nursing home social worker, who met with her weekly and helped her sort out her ambivalent feelings toward her daughter. Gradually, Grace made a few friends among the other residents and found she could enjoy discussion groups, ceramics, and even bingo with the other women on her floor.

Grace Fitzgerald may have been a victim of the current trend toward romanticization of home life. Home conjures up the image of a large old house, filled with family heirlooms and photographs, a house that has been in the family for decades and perhaps continues to be inhabited by several generations. Grandma is cheerfully ensconced in her own room, doted on by her loving daughter and entertained by the apples of her eye, her young grandchildren. Other family members are constantly dropping in, so there is always someone available to spend time with Grandma. The grandmother in this idyll wears glasses and a hearing-aid, and uses a cane (itself a family heirloom) to get around. She has trouble with constipation and is a bit forgetful, but she is basically in that group which I have called the robust elderly. The reality, unfortunately, is often quite different.

Perhaps the most fundamental reason this portrait of graceful aging is so seldom accurate is that life expectancy has increased. Life expectancy at birth is 70.9 years for men and 78.2 years for women. More important, for those who survive to retirement age, life expectancy is 14.5 years for men and 18.8 years for women.[8] This translates into a population as of 1986 in which there are 2.8 million people over 80 and 25,000 people who are over 100.[9] With the tremendous growth of the so-called "old old" has come a more prolonged period of disability.[10] An older population, quite simply, means a greater probability of physical dependence: while only 15 percent of community-dwelling elders aged 65–69 need help with the activities of daily living, that percentage shoots up to 49 percent in individuals over 85.[11] An older population also means a rising risk of dementia, with one community survey reporting a prevalence as high as 47 percent in people over 85.[12] Between mental impairment and physical dependence, there are not that many very elderly people who can make do with family merely looking in.

The second factor affecting the frequency with which old people live with family is, of course, the waning of the extended family. Although family members continue to provide the bulk of caretaking for the elderly—80 percent in some reports,[13] or an average of four hours a day[14]—the mobility of Americans has led to the dispersion of the family. There often is no one living in the same city as the old person, let alone in the same house. And when there is a son or a daughter in the vicinity, that adult child is often employed (65 percent of adult women aged 45–54 now work outside the home)[15] or is herself elderly and may be unable to provide a great deal of assistance.

The majority of elderly people clearly prefer home to institutional living. But for many, home is a small apartment, perhaps in senior citizen housing. It may be structurally inadequate: a person with bilateral amputations is not going to thrive in a second floor walkup with a bathroom that is too small to be wheelchair-accessible. It may be isolating—remote from shopping, away from friends, without social activities on the premises. Finally, as with Grace Fitzgerald, home can be a difficult setting in which to obtain adequate caretaking. Grace's situation was far from unique: since homemakers and home health aides are unskilled, uneducated, poorly paid, and often unsupervised, they may as easily prove to be disastrous as life-saving.[16]

The move toward keeping the chronically ill elderly at home also reflects the dreadful reputation of nursing homes. Several landmark muckraking works[17] have helped to bring many profound deficiencies of nursing homes to light. Good journalism has disclosed financial scandals in which vulnerable old people were neglected while nursing home chain owners reaped a profit. The abuses in nursing homes were, and continue to be, very real: nursing home residents are sometimes excessively sedated with antipsychotic medications;[18] medical care is often cursory or shoddy;[19] the autonomy and independence of residents are routinely ignored;[20] aides are too few to keep the residents dry and clean; residents are often restrained in geri-chairs, special chairs with a tray that serves to prevent the person from getting out of the chair, with little or no social stimulation.[21]

Increasing scrutiny of nursing homes through a federal ombudsman program, tightening government regulation of nursing homes, and growing academic interest in improving the quality of nursing homes by developing community teaching nursing homes have led to the elimination of many substandard homes and the creation of some outstanding ones. An extensive investigation of nursing homes, culminating in a report issued in 1986 by the Institute of Medicine[22] (many of whose recommendations were incorporated into federal law), has set higher standards for nursing homes.

The poor reputation of nursing homes, however, derives from more than a sometimes sordid reality. Institutional long-term care is feared and loathed because of a long tradition of regarding nursing homes as places of last resort, shelters for the destitute. The ancestor of the contemporary American nursing home is the nineteenth-century almshouse, a refuge for paupers. Residents of an almshouse were stigmatized as misfits, individuals who had ostensibly brought poverty and disability upon themselves.[23] Only the most abject entered an almshouse in the nineteenth century. The older American today often believes that only people who were too incompetent to make provisions for their old age or too disagreeable to have a caring family could possibly end up in a nursing home.

There is an institutional alternative to nursing home care today, the board and care facility, which arose in the nineteenth century as an alternative to the almshouse for the "respectable poor."[24] These are small homes, designed as residences for elderly people who need some assistance with personal care and who are unable to do their own housekeeping. Because they are not considered medical institutions, they are not covered by Medicaid and can serve exclusively a privately paying clientele. At rates of eighty, ninety, or even a hundred dollars a day, there are not many people who can afford such facilities. In certified skilled nursing homes, the vast majority of residents who enter paying privately have "spent down" all their resources by the end of six months of institutionalization; at this point, Medicaid is available to pick up the tab. No such option is available in the homier board and care facilities. For Grace Fitzgerald, who had already used up most of what savings she had on personal care attendants, a board and care home was out of the question. She was fortunate that Silver Days was able to preserve a bit of the flavor of an old-fashioned home by grouping the mentally intact residents together, permitting a few personal furnishings, and offering engaging social activities.

Once Grace was in a protected environment, her medical problems readily came under control. The goals of medical care for her were comfort always, maintenance of function whenever possible, and cure if the recommended treatment was not excessively disruptive to her precarious equilibrium. She intuitively recognized what Sam Schaeffer had not appreciated: that she had far less tolerance for medical interventions than her more robust counterparts. She learned the hard way that her symptoms were sometimes as likely to be affected by non-medical interventions, such as moving to the nursing home, as by conventional medical treatment. Are there any frail individuals for whom virtually all standard medical therapy is excessively burdensome, in whom only personal care and modifications of the environment are warranted? Or is there some minimum level of medical care that is in the best interest of every patient, no matter how frail? I was forced to confront these questions when I returned from a visit to Grace Fitzgerald at Silver Days to find a frantic message on my desk. A surgeon at the hospital wanted urgently to speak with me. He had a fairly unusual request: he wanted me to take over the care of one of his patients.

The Best Interest of the Patient

When her friends and family described Margaret Chadwick, they always came around to saying how determined she was. Her closest college friend recalled how determined Margaret had been to persuade the administration of her college to invite a distinguished woman graduate to speak at commencement. College graduation had come just at the end of World War II, when women had discovered that they could do almost anything men could do and were sought after for all sorts of jobs in the men's absence, only to find upon the soldiers' return that they were now expected to retreat into the home and free up all the jobs for the men. Margaret Chadwick believed that women should decide for themselves whether they wished to stay home or go to work, and not have that decision made by men. She was determined that her classmates should have at least one role model of a woman who had graduated from their college and then gone on to have a successful career as a distinguished law professor. Margaret argued and complained and insisted until finally she had her way.

It was determination that led to the birth of the Chadwicks' daughter, Anne. Margaret married Henry Chadwick when she was 30, and when they subsequently decided to have a child, they ran into difficulty. Three miscarriages later, Margaret's physician advised the couple to adopt, saying that she was simply too old to carry a baby to term. This was before the era of infertility specialists and of neonatal intensive care units in which 26-week-old preemies could be salvaged. Margaret was determined to have her own biological child, however. Since she had successfully carried a child for six and a half months, she reasoned, the reproductive apparatus was basically working. If only she could maintain the pregnancy for a few extra weeks, things might turn out fine. She went to a nearby medical library and discovered data suggesting that bedrest might prevent miscarriages in the third trimester.

At age 38, after six years of effort and five miscarriages, Margaret Chadwick gave birth to a normal baby girl. She was born six weeks early, weighing in at 4½ pounds. Margaret had spent ten weeks at virtually complete bedrest, waited upon by her husband. Baby Anne spent a few weeks in the hospital in an incubator. When the doctors satisfied themselves that her lungs were sufficiently mature for her to breathe properly, and her liver was sufficiently mature to prevent jaundice, she was sent home. Once home, Anne developed like any other baby, requiring no special medical attention.

When Margaret Chadwick turned 60, she developed diabetes. There was a strong family history of diabetes, and Margaret had always been careful to stay thin and avoid sweets. Despite her efforts, her pancreas produced less and less of the insulin necessary to regulate blood sugar levels, and within two years of diagnosis, Margaret had gone from controlling the disease by diet alone, to using oral medication, to injecting insulin.

At age 65, Margaret had her first heart attack. As often happens with diabetics, she had none of the classical signs: she had no crushing chest pain, no pain radiating into her left arm, no sweats or nausea. She woke up feeling vaguely ill one morning and thought she was coming down with the flu. When she tried to make the bed and set the table for breakfast, she found herself short of breath. Margaret went back to bed, having long ago decided that bedrest was the cure for most ailments, and would have stayed there had she not developed an odd pain in her neck and jaw. Her daughter Anne, who by then was a psychiatric nurse, chanced to telephone, and when she heard her mother's symptoms, insisted that her mother see her physician immediately. Margaret was found to be in mild congestive heart failure—her lungs were filling with fluid from an inadequately pumping heart—and an electrocardiogram disclosed that she was having a heart attack.

Margaret had recovered uneventfully from the heart attack when she noticed she was developing leg cramps every time she walked a block or more. She was found to have peripheral vascular disease—atherosclerosis involving the arteries to her legs, caused most likely by diabetes and high blood pressure. For the first time Margaret had to cut back on her usual activities, not just for a brief period, as when she had been hospitalized with the heart attack, but for good. She could no longer go on walks along the beach at the family vacation cottage on Martha's Vineyard: her legs would not let her. She could no longer garden in her backyard: she got chest pain and shortness of breath from lack of oxygen to her heart. She took half a dozen different medications for her heart as well as insulin for her diabetes, and found that she could function well within her home and could travel if she was taken door-to-door. Margaret began to write letters to friends whom she could no longer visit with any degree of frequency. She had long telephone conversations with her daughter and began, in her voluminous spare time, to keep a diary.

The gist of Margaret's letters, her diary entries, and her conversations was that she was determined not to keep on living if she became unable to take care of herself, if she could not communicate, if she could not recognize her family. She no longer believed that she could successfully vanquish her diabetes and vascular disease. She did, however, think that she could control the kind of medical care she would receive in the future.

One heart attack later, Margaret Chadwick found that the pumping function of her heart was sufficiently impaired that she tired quickly even within her own home. She could not walk from one room to another without getting leg cramps. Fortunately, her husband, although thirteen years her senior, was a spry 80-year-old who was able to do all the shopping and housework for the two of them. In addition, her daughter Anne lived a mere twenty miles away and was able to come weekly to help out and, more important, to talk. It was during one of these visits that Margaret indicated that she felt she was living with just about as much disability as she could tolerate. If she sustained any further blows, she would not want her life preserved.

The next blow came a month later. Margaret developed a cold, blue, excruciatingly painful left leg. She went to the hospital in search of relief from the pain, and was found to have thrown a blood clot from her heart to a blood vessel in her leg, totally blocking off the circulation. She was put on heparin to help dissolve the clot and prevent further clots. The doctors talked about operating, though Margaret made it very clear that she did not want surgery unless the heparin afforded her no relief. While the debate continued, Margaret had a massive stroke.

A computerized tomographic (CT) scan of the head demonstrated that she had bled into her brain. Longstanding high blood pressure, only moderately well controlled, put her at high risk for just such a bleed. Perhaps the heparin had been the final straw. In any event, one afternoon when Margaret's nurse entered her room to take routine temperature, pulse, and blood pressure readings, she found her paralyzed on the right side, unable to speak, and very lethargic.

Over the next two weeks, Margaret became less sleepy but remained incapable of uttering a single coherent word. Her right arm and leg were lifeless. She followed people with her eyes but showed no sign of recognition when her husband or daughter entered the room. She could obey simple commands such as "close your eyes," albeit inconsistently. Occasionally she cried; rarely she smiled.

During those two weeks following the stroke, Margaret had two CT scans (the initial one and a follow-up), a brainwave test or electroencephalogram, daily blood drawing to monitor her blood sugars, daily physical therapy, speech therapy and occupational therapy, and consultations by a neurologist, a psychiatrist, and an internist. The neurologist confirmed that the brain damage was extensive and the prognosis poor, but stated that the full extent of recovery of function, if any, would not be known for weeks, perhaps months. The psychiatrist acknowledged that Margaret had been rendered incapable of making health and safety decisions for herself. The three therapists reported that they had detected no progress in two weeks; moreover, Margaret's inability to comprehend instructions rendered her a poor candidate for further rehabilitative efforts.

To Anne and Henry, the situation was clear-cut. Margaret had had a devastating stroke. She had had intensive treatment for two weeks and showed no signs of improvement. Although she could conceivably make some slight degree of progress in the future, "progress" meant a few scattered words, maybe an occasional phrase, a flicker of movement in her fingers. To call this progress struck Margaret's family as ludicrous. Anything less than the restoration of language and mobility was hopelessly inadequate. Sitting mindlessly in a chair, unable to feed herself, incontinent, Margaret was viewed by her husband and daughter—and they felt certain she would have viewed herself in this way—as trapped in a condition worse than death. Under the circumstances, the family agreed, Margaret would want to be kept comfortable. She would not wish to be given any medication, whether blood pressure pills or medication against angina, whose goal was to prevent further strokes or heart attacks and thus to prolong life. They therefore asked Margaret's physician to discontinue all medications that were not explicitly and unambiguously devoted to amelioration of suffering. They wished intravenous fluids to be discontinued, insisting that she be spoon-fed and that her nutrition and hydration be limited to whatever she was able to take by mouth.

To Margaret's physician, the situation was also clear-cut. Margaret was not terminally ill: her vascular disease was severe and progressive, but with treatment of her blood pressure and her diabetes it probably would not kill her in the next six months. She was not in a persistent vegetative state: she had a good deal more brain function than Karen Quinlan or Nancy Cruzan had had. Therefore, her doctor believed, she had no medical condition that justified the limitation or withdrawal of medical treatment. Dr. Richardson, the surgeon who was in charge of Margaret's case, was very blunt. Failing to give Margaret antihypertensive medication and halting the intravenous fluids would be tantamount to killing her.

Meetings between Dr. Richardson and Margaret's family became increasingly acrimonious. The hospital social worker and the chaplain were unsuccessful in their attempts to mediate. Ultimately, as usually happens in cases of irreconcilable disagreement, Henry and Anne Chadwick went to court to obtain guardianship of Margaret.

They succeeded not only in becoming co-guardians, but in obtaining specific court authorization for the withdrawal of all medications except insulin, which was viewed by the judge as replacing a natural bodily substance rather than as a treatment for disease. Dr. Richardson, extremely dismayed by what he regarded as the court dictating medical treatment to him, sought another doctor to take over the case.

I became, at this charged and tragic moment in Margaret Chadwick's life, her doctor. When I went to see Margaret, I found a moderately obese woman propped up in a chair, her hair only slightly gray. She looked young to me, perhaps because I am so used to patients in their eighties that a 67-year-old appeared youthful. Her right arm lay motionless on her lap, like something foreign, alien. Her left arm was curled around a plump brown teddy bear with a red ribbon around its neck. Her eyes followed me as I came over to her. I told her who I was, I asked her how she felt. Her face remained expressionless. I tried talking to her for a while, referring to my telephone conversation with her daughter, commenting that she had been through a great deal. She watched me at first, then shifted her gaze to the teddy bear, and then, as I began examining her, she fell asleep.

It was difficult to withhold treatment from Margaret Chadwick both because she was not dying and because of the uncertainty surrounding her prognosis. The evidence I had available suggested that the likelihood of Margaret's achieving a recovery significant enough to her to warrant further life-prolonging interventions was vanishingly small. She had only barely been functioning at a level she deemed satisfactory before the stroke. Unless she recovered fully, which was virtually certain not to happen, she would not have wanted further medical treatment. Anne and Henry's account of Margaret's goals in life, of what was important to her, and of her expressed wishes, substantiated in large measure by her letters and diaries, led me to believe that Margaret would not have wanted to be given medications except to make her comfortable.

In accordance with the guardians' wishes, as explicitly authorized by the court, I ordered that Margaret be fed to the extent that she could tolerate food and drink, and that all pills be stopped. She continued to receive her usual dose of insulin. Anti-anginal medications were to be stopped unless they were needed to treat chest pain. No further blood tests were to be performed. Intravenous fluids were discontinued. None of these measures led to Margaret's death. Her blood pressure rose, but otherwise there was no discernible effect of the discontinuation of the medications. Clearly, the utility of the medication had been primarily to prevent future, long-term vascular events (strokes and heart attacks), not to sustain daily life.

Three days later, Margaret Chadwick died. She died from complications of her stroke, not from the withholding of her usual medicines. Because her swallowing mechanism was impaired, some of the food she was given went into her lungs instead of her stomach. This gave her a pneumonitis, an inflammation of the lungs resulting from food that was in the wrong place. She quickly developed a high fever, dehydration, and a rapid respiratory rate. Her blood pressure began to fall; she lost consciousness; and she died peacefully.

The surgeon caring for Margaret Chadwick had been reluctant

to treat her in accordance with her family's wishes because of the widespread reluctance to limit medical treatment for someone who is not terminally ill. Margaret was not terminally ill in the conventional sense of having a uniformly fatal condition with a life expectancy of less than six months. Her underlying atherosclerosis was progressive, but hardly certain to kill her in short order. The reason for the family's request to limit care was not the relentless atherosclerosis, but rather the devastation wrought by a single episode of bleeding into the brain. Not only was Margaret Chadwick not terminally ill; she was neither in a coma nor in a persistent vegetative state. Unlike Karen Quinlan, who remained comatose, unresponsive to any stimuli, from the time of her overdose from alcohol and tranquilizers in 1975 to her demise ten years later, and unlike Nancy Cruzan, whose eyes roamed vacantly, unseeing and unfeeling seven years after an automobile accident, Margaret Chadwick was awake and could respond to voice and to touch. She did not have a degenerative disease such as Alzheimer's disease, which would result in her gradual deterioration over a period of years. Margaret simply did not fit into a neat little box labeled coma or persistent vegetative state or terminal illness or Alzheimer's disease. And yet she had suffered a tremendous blow which undermined her remaining physical and mental capacity.

Because Margaret had lost such a great deal of her much-vaunted independence, with no prospect that even her legendary determination would bring about a significant amelioration of her condition, her family felt that the goal of her medical care should become comfort rather than cure. Since there was no cure for her stroke, they saw little purpose in seeking to cure other comparatively minor ailments such as infections. Unlike Claire Renan, however, they did not demand euthanasia. They understood that Margaret could conceivably linger for months, paralyzed, unable to speak, comprehending only intermittently and then merely the simplest of phrases. What Henry and Anne did request was that I discontinue the numerous pills Margaret had been taking to control her blood pressure and to prevent angina, which they regarded as superfluous, given her condition.

While mentally competent individuals have a well-established ethical and legal right to refuse any medical treatment,[25] surrogates for patients incapable of making their own health care decisions typically seek only to withhold or withdraw life-sustaining care, usually in the setting of coma, persistent vegetative state, or terminal illness. The kind of medical care that Henry and Anne Chadwick sought to limit was routine, everyday treatment that could hardly be construed as invasive, aggressive, or intrusive.

Distinctions between "extraordinary" and "ordinary" care have largely fallen out of favor, since what seems like a heroic measure to one person may appear quite commonplace to another.[26] Thus, ventilator support can be withdrawn or withheld not because it is extraordinary care, but rather because it is life-sustaining treatment that may pointlessly prolong the dying process of a hopelessly ill individual. The U.S. Supreme Court has endorsed the concept that all medical treatments are created equal: distinguishing between different kinds of interventions is simply not meaningful. The administration of artificial nutrition and hydration, the Court concluded in its only right-to-die case to date, the Cruzan case, is a medical treatment and therefore, like all other medical treatments, can be withdrawn or withheld from patients at their request or by their representatives. The Justices were clearly troubled by the question of whether there should be any restrictions on the power of surrogate decision makers. Were there any clinical conditions in which limiting care was inappropriate? Were there any kinds of care that could not be limited? The Court resolved this by affirming that individual state legislatures could place a major restriction on surrogate decision making: they could require that surrogates adduce clear and convincing evidence that the proposed limitations were in accordance with the patient's previously stated wishes.[27] In short, had Margaret Chadwick lived in Missouri or New York, the two states which have passed such laws, Henry and Anne would have had difficulty demanding that I stop her medications. Margaret's diary, her correspondence, and her family's recollections of their conversations with her all pointed to her regarding life after a major stroke as intolerable. However, they did not conclusively demonstrate just exactly what she would have wanted done in the event of a stroke, and they certainly conveyed no specific instructions about pill-taking.

Margaret Chadwick lived in the state of Massachusetts when she was hospitalized with a cold blue leg and then went on to develop a massive intracerebral hemorrhage. In Massachusetts the major legal precedent is the Brophy case, in which Paul Brophy's family petitioned for the cessation of artificial nutrition and hydration after he sustained another kind of cerebral hemorrhage: a subarachnoid bleed in which a small outpouching or aneurysm of one of the arteries of the brain, a defect in the lining of the blood vessel, abruptly burst, spilling blood into the cavity surrounding the brain. Paul Brophy lost consciousness after surgery designed to prevent further leaks. When, after two years, he had not woken up, and multiple neurologists confirmed his grim prognosis, his devoutly Catholic family felt enough was enough. They recalled that Mr. Brophy, a firefighter with copious experience with catastrophe, had stated that he would want the plug pulled if he were ever in a condition like that of Karen Quinlan. The Massachusetts Supreme Judicial Court upheld the right of the family to authorize the withdrawal of any medical treatment, including artificial nutrition and fluid. The family, it was presumed, was in the best position to know what Paul Brophy would have wanted for himself.[28] The Brophy family was not required to prove beyond the shadow of a doubt that their relative in fact would have declined a feeding tube, had he known he would be in a vegetative state. Likewise, the Chadwick family was assumed to be in the best position to accept or reject medical treatments for Margaret.

Suppose Margaret Chadwick had been in excruciating pain—if,

for example, the heparin had been unsuccessful in dissolving the clot in her leg. And suppose further that Henry and Anne had insisted that the surgeon give no pain medication. Would that have been an acceptable decision? Are there truly no limits on surrogate decision-making power outside of those states with specific laws controlling the circumstances in which they may act?

There are limits on surrogate decision making, just as there are limits on what patients can choose for themselves. Patients cannot demand treatment for which there is no demonstrable efficacy: professionalism requires that physicians do *not* prescribe penicillin for viral infections or laetrile for breast cancer or vitamins for ear infections.[29] Moreover, if patients refuse treatment that most patients would accept, physicians are obligated to ascertain why they are refusing. Their right to refuse is qualified: they need to be able to give a coherent justification for seemingly irrational behavior.[30] Not only must patients be clearly capable of making decisions—understanding the nature of the proposed therapy, its anticipated effect, and the consequences of refusing therapy[31]—but patients' refusal must also be consistent with their values. Otherwise patients might refuse lifesaving treatment because of a misapprehension of fact: they might decline surgery because of an erroneous belief that it would result in impotence or in intractable postoperative pain.

Since seemingly intact, competent patients cannot simply refuse generally accepted medical treatment without explanation, then surely surrogates cannot decline medical care on behalf of others without careful questioning of the basis for their request.[32] If the Chadwicks had asked that Margaret not be given pain medication for extreme pain in her leg, the surgeon would have been within his rights to find out their rationale. Unless they had supplied proof that Margaret had specifically and consistently stated that she never under any circumstances wished to have pain medication, the surgeon would have had good reason to deny their request, to challenge their right to serve as surrogates, and in fact to file a claim against them for elder abuse. Indeed, even if Margaret Chadwick had resolutely refused narcotics in the past, the surgeon would have been entitled to ask why. If the reason had been a fear of addiction, he would have been able to reassure her family that addiction was not a realistic concern at this juncture in her life.

When I agreed to take over Margaret Chadwick's care, it was because I was satisfied that Henry and Anne were articulating very reasonable goals for Margaret. They had no ulterior motives in requesting that the various medications be discontinued. A judge had ruled that there was sufficient evidence to conclude that Margaret Chadwick, had she been able to speak for herself, would have wanted only supportive care. But the truth was that there was only indirect evidence about what exactly Margaret would or would not have wanted. She had been explicit that if her heart stopped, she did not wish to be resuscitated. She had been fairly clear that she would not want to spend the remainder of her life on a respirator. She had said many times that her life, even before the stroke, was only barely tolerable, implying that she could not imagine adjusting to further deficits. But she most decidedly had not said anything about what kind of medical care she would want if she developed new medical problems.

The only way that Henry and Anne, or the judge, or I as her physician, could decide whether to withhold antihypertensive and anti-anginal medications from Margaret Chadwick was on the basis of an assessment of her best interests. Our view was that what was best for Margaret Chadwick was no different from what was best for any patient in her condition, and was very much analogous to what was best for patients with dementia. Even though the basis of her cognitive deficits was a stroke rather than Alzheimer's disease, she was reduced to a very similar condition. Her concomitant physical deficits merely made her situation an order of magnitude worse: unlike Maria Londino in the early stages of dementia, she could not walk down the corridor and enjoy the sights. Anne and Henry petitioned for the discontinuation of Margaret's medications because they sensed that the goal of treatment for anyone in her condition should be to relieve pain and maintain dignity. Margaret's long-standing personality traits—her fierce independence and her determination—and her prior comments that her life was nearly intolerable even before the stroke only strengthened their resolve.

There are limits to what families can reasonably be allowed to refuse, just as there are limits to what families can reasonably be allowed to demand. Tony Londino, in requesting hospital-level care for his severely demented mother, exceeded what most individuals intimately aware of their respective situations would have regarded as appropriate and humane. His request was nonetheless honored out of respect for proxy decision making. The Chadwicks came perilously close to demanding that more be withheld from Margaret than most physicians would deem acceptable.

If reasonable goals of treatment for the robust elderly are life-prolongation and cure, if reasonable goals for the demented elderly are maximization of function and palliation, and if the overriding goal for the dying is achievement of comfort, what are the corresponding goals for the frail elderly? Defining a single goal of medical care is problematic. Instead, there should be upper and lower bounds to what constitutes appropriate treatment in this group: an upper bound based on the kinds of intervention frail patients are able to tolerate, and a lower bound based on the best interests of even the frailest of patients. For Sam Schaeffer, maximally aggressive therapy was predictably disastrous. An alternative approach would have made far more sense, not because Mr. Schaeffer's quality of life was too poor to merit vigorous treatment, but rather because his body was too weak to withstand the onslaught of medicine's most heavily armored battalions. For Margaret Chadwick, the goal of treatment was maintenance of comfort. Her family chose to limit her care on the basis of their assessment of what was appropriate for someone in her condition, tempered by what she would have wanted. But they were not entitled to demand that more be withheld than was consistent with providing Mrs. Chadwick a minimum standard of care. In selecting goals of treatment between these boundaries, frail older people and their representatives need to understand not only the perils of both overtreatment and undertreatment, but also the limited role of medical interventions in determining their quality of life. Clearly medical care has much to offer, but the role of nontechnical factors, such as a nursing home for a patient like Grace Fitzgerald, can be just as important.

❖ 5 ❖

The Means to the Ends: Institutional Changes

By the time most of my elderly patients become frail, and almost certainly by the time they are dying, they have come to accept their own mortality. They may not like it, as was the case with Madeleine Kane, an elegant, dignified woman in her nineties dying of metastatic breast cancer. I recall her grabbing my hand urgently, telling me: "I don't want to die." But even she, while frightened of dying, frightened of experiencing pain and of being alone, even she understood and accepted the inevitability of death. My older patients may hope desperately that I can prolong their lives just a bit, as did Mary Soloway, who told me with tears in her eyes that she wanted to live to see the birth of her twelfth great-grandchild. She lay in the coronary care unit after her third heart attack and was adamant that she would not consider angioplasty to open up her clogged arteries, and she certainly would not contemplate bypass surgery. She understood that she was already on every available cardiac medication, from beta blockers to reduce her heart's workload, to anticoagulants to keep her blood from clotting in the narrow arteries leading to her heart, to calcium channel blockers to prevent angina through their effect on ion flows within the heart tissue. She fully comprehended that if she did not accept angioplasty or a bypass, she in all probability would not live to see her new great-grandchild. She knew this; she simply wished it were not so.

Those who have the most difficulty accepting the limits of medicine's ability to prolong life are often the family members of elderly patients. Florence Arzmanian was one of my house call patients. While hospitalized for chest pain, she was found to have a tumor filling up a large part of her left lung. Tests of her sputum proved the tumor to be malignant. Given her age, her heart condition, and her other underlying medical problems such as emphysema, she was not an operative candidate. The chest surgeon and the oncologist who examined her agreed that palliation with radiation therapy, in the hope of improving her breathing and her chest pain, was the best option. Mrs. Arzmanian agreed, saying forcefully that she did not want an operation. She understood that without surgery she would die, but she also understood that with surgery she could die too, and probably sooner. Mrs. Arzmanian's daughter was not nearly as sanguine. "You mean you aren't going to do anything? You're just going to let her die?" she asked in disbelief. I tried to reassure her that there was a great deal we were doing: radiation therapy would help to shrink the tumor, and when the time came, we could give her oxygen and ample pain medication to prevent her from suffering. Mrs. Arzmanian's daughter seemed a bit reassured, but still skeptical. The next day I had a telephone call from a second daughter, who was equally incredulous. How was it possible, she wanted to know, that there could be a disease without a cure?

Here were two women, themselves in their sixties, who simply could not accept the fact that their 95-year-old mother would not live forever. Nor were they unique. Tony Londino had tremendous difficulty letting go, even when his mother's demented existence was finally coming to an end thanks to a massive heart attack. Sam Schaeffer's daughter, who encouraged her father to opt for valve replacement surgery rather than for the simpler but often not curative valvuloplasty, pushed for the definitive operation because she thought of the body as a machine, each of whose failing parts could be replaced without any inherent limit to longevity. There are, of course, plenty of families who do accept the inevitability of death. Jennie Rosetti's son understood full well, as Jennie lay intubated in the intensive care unit, that one organ system after another was giving way, and that there was no point trying vainly to stave off death. Margaret Chadwick's husband and daughter recognized even before her devastating stroke that she was living the final chapter of her life. With her heart attacks, her longstanding diabetes, and her severe peripheral vascular disease, it was just a question of how to write the denouement.

Although some families are realistic about what to expect from their aging relatives, many Americans have little conception of what aging entails and are unaccepting of the ultimate reality of death. Despite the attention accorded death and dying by the work of Elisabeth Kubler-Ross,[1] death is still hidden from the view of most families. Very few people actually die at home anymore. Fully 61 percent of Americans over 65 who die do so in the hospital, and another 22 percent die in nursing homes, leaving only 17 percent of the 1,465,896 annual deaths to take place at home.[2]

Perhaps even more disturbing than the lack of familiarity with death is the widespread expectation that people will remain vigorous and healthy until, abruptly, they die. This is the image of aging that is perpetuated by magazines targeted to the older person; it is the myth that forms the basis for a whole slew of self-help books that are meant to keep people well as they age; and it is the model of aging embodied in our health care system, which reimburses for acute medical care but is severely deficient in its approach to chronic care.

A random sample of the fare served up by America's premier magazine for the older retired person conveys a world radically different from the reality that confronted Maria Londino, Margaret Chadwick, or Sam Schaeffer. The feature articles suggest that the typical older person is able and eager to continue working[3] as well as to sustain interests in film, music, and literature.[4] A regular travelogue department plus abundant advertisements for dream vacations bolster the idea that the elderly will be vigorous enough to travel extensively in their retirement years. Most disconcerting of all, the advertisements present a portrait of today's senior citizens as individuals of considerable means who will remain healthy if only they eat enough fiber, avoid salt and caffeine, keep their cholesterol down, and take a vitamin supplement. They may want to use special skin creams to remain beautiful, but the only assistive devices mentioned are a "clean-up" machine for the garden and an electric scooter for transportation from the bridge club to the dining hall of a prestigious residential retirement community, not walkers or canes. While many elderly individuals are indeed robust, as were Panos Pappadokoulos, Rebecca Landsman, and Joseph Kohlman (at least until they became ill and inched their way toward frailty), there is a conspicuous absence of anybody who is demented, frail, or dying from the magazine's pages. Occasionally a reader will complain, as in one letter to the editor commenting: "My siblings and I are tired of the bouncing, hyperactive 'seniors' pictured in your paper … Life is not all that blissful when you hit the mid-70s. Engines knock and wheels wobble."[5]

A host of self-help books have appeared over the past decade that are similarly devoted to the belief that aging is something to be conquered, or at least subdued, and that with a good attitude and a good diet, there is no such thing as frailty. Books such as *Your Vitality Quotient: The Clinically Proven Program That Can Reduce Your Body Age and Increase Your Zest for Life*[6] and *Forever Young: 20 Years Younger in 20 Weeks: Dr. Berger's Step-by-Step Rejuvenating Program*[7] suggest not merely that aging is avoidable, but also that it is reversible. Other how-to manuals subscribe to the theory that most people can "expect to live heartily, fully, with all functions intact, into the 80s" and then abruptly pass away.[8] These authors tout, in addition to diet and exercise, intellectual stimulation, social interaction, sex, and sleep. They also subscribe to the view that if people would only express their emotions instead of keeping their feelings bottled up inside and if they had faith of some kind, whether in God, in a life force, in humanity, or in themselves, they would suffer no disease or disability in old age.[9]

There is, of course, a role for diet and exercise in maintaining health and well-being. Diet is the treatment of choice for adult onset diabetes, a major risk factor for heart disease in the elderly and a cause of impaired vision and kidney failure. Exercise can prevent obesity, a major contributing factor to arthritis, and specific strengthening exercises can improve the ability of people even in their nineties to walk and to carry bundles.[10] The view of aging as a time of inevitably declining physical and mental health is as flawed as the view of aging as the golden years. Many of the disabilities so common in Western society are unheard-of in other cultures, calling into serious question the assumption that American-style aging is synonymous with normal aging.[11] Activity is clearly superior to a sedentary existence, and diets low in fat, salt, and sweets are undeniably preferable to those loaded with cholesterol, salt, and sugar. But Margaret Chadwick developed diabetes despite fastidious attention to diet. Her diabetes was in all likelihood genetically determined, since she had a strong family history of diabetes. Her high blood pressure, too, ran in the family and was beyond her control. And it was the combination of diabetes and high blood pressure which led to her heart attacks, which caused the impaired circulation in her legs, and which predisposed her to a stroke. Her condition would probably have been worse if Margaret had not meticulously followed her prescribed diet, monitored her insulin carefully, and pushed herself to work in the garden and walk on the beach as long as possible. But to blame Margaret Chadwick for her frailty—to suppose that if only she had taken greater control of her life, she would have diminished her disabilities—is a gross misunderstanding of the vagaries of human destiny.

If frailty is often unavoidable, so too is dementia. The magazine *Modern Maturity* advertises products to help older adults improve their memory; *Conquest of Aging* asserts that "a very large percentage of memory 'defects' in the long-lived are curable, almost all are improvable," goes on to claim that "memory skills can be learned at any age," and finally concludes that "the recuperative powers of the human mind, particularly when enhanced by specific training, are far more extensive than most people believe."[12] The key to the prevention and treatment of dementia lies in research laboratories that are working on understanding the molecular basis of Alzheimer's disease;[13] it lies in clinical trials of medication which, on the basis of fundamental biological research, is thought to offer some promise.[14] It does not lie in memory enhancement exercises or in flagrant denial that there is a problem, as when a 750-page reference book about aging devotes one paragraph to "senile dementia."[15] Maria Londino and Nadine Chang led exemplary lives. There was nothing they could have done to prevent the onslaught of Alzheimer's disease, and once the dementia hit with full force, no brain-stretching activities could reverse the tide. This is not to imply that interventions failed to make a difference in their lives. Tony's painstaking care of his mother permitted her to remain at home, in a familiar environment, much longer than would otherwise have been feasible. His advocacy for his mother when she finally did enter a nursing home, though a perpetual source of irritation for the nursing staff, most likely did serve to keep the staff on their toes, more attentive to the little things that profoundly affected Maria's quality of life. Mrs. Chang likewise was stricken with a relentlessly progressive dementing illness. Neither right eating nor right thinking could have expanded her vocabulary beyond "bababa" or enabled her to recognize her family. A gentle and dedicated live-in caretaker, however, made a tremendous difference in her life by dressing and bathing her with infinite tenderness and patience.

If dementia and frailty are frequent concomitants of aging, and illness is an almost invariable feature of getting old, death is the culmination of the aging process. The simple truth is that we all die eventually, and those who are fortunate enough to survive to old age are rapidly approaching the end of the road. Once we acknowledge that we will all die, the issue becomes not so much when, and certainly not whether, but rather what path to take.

Which road to choose, what approach to take in treating the medical problems of the elderly, depends on the burdens and benefits of treatment. Contemporary American bioethicists suggest that this measuring of risks and benefits is an entirely individual, subjective process. Each person who develops a medical problem, according to this view, should be presented with the available options for treatment and should choose a course of therapy based on an understanding of the pros and cons of each possibility and on careful introspection, a soul-searching examination of personal values. I have argued that while there is a role for personal preference—some people may be more risk-averse than others, or have a higher tolerance for pain or suffering—the importance of individual preferences has been overrated.

If reasonable people face the issues head on—if we acknowledge that we will all die, if we recognize that those of us fortunate enough to make it to old age will develop disease and disability, and if we consider the possible ways of responding to disease—we will recognize that we can define appropriate goals of treatment, goals that should vary depending on whether the patient is robust, demented, dying, or frail. For the robust, the appropriate goal in general is cure, prolonging life, much as in younger people. For the demented, the goal should be maximizing function. Care is palliative and rehabilitative. It can be curative provided this is not excessively grueling. For the dying, the most reasonable goal is comfort. Treatment is supportive. Sometimes life-sustaining treatment is warranted as the best way to ensure comfort: for example, a painful and dangerous abscess should be opened and drained; it may be reasonable to treat pneumonia with antibiotics and oxygen as the best means to prevent a patient from gasping for breath. For frail patients, the goal of medical care should be cure when possible, recognizing that these individuals have such a poor tolerance for interventions that often cure is not realistically feasible. When the price of curative therapy is prohibitive, maximization of function becomes the more plausible goal. And in the frailest of the frail, in whom functioning is already extremely tenuous, only comfort is a realistic goal.

What makes these goals of medical treatment reasonable? The goals emerge as humane and attainable because they derive not merely from an evaluation of the quality of life of aging individuals before the onset of acute illness, and not merely from an acceptance of human mortality, but also from an understanding of what the treatment of disease actually entails. My argument is that even without the benefit of careful, philosophical analysis, the vast majority of people, when confronted with the nature of the experience of illness, will agree on the reasonableness of these goals.[16]

Within this framework there remain ample opportunities for individual choice. There is choice; simply not unlimited choice. The frail or demented elderly should not be asked whether they would like to have cardiopulmonary resuscitation attempted if their hearts stop beating. The dying elderly should not be asked whether they wish dialysis if, in the course of dying from metastatic cancer, their kidneys fail. But the robust elderly certainly have the choice to forgo dialysis, as did Matilda Burney. They can choose to undergo a colectomy, as did Rebecca Landsman, despite being 95, because it was, in her view, the best way to obtain relief from her symptoms. Older individuals or their surrogates need to start with prescribed goals, and then take the broad outlines of what would constitute a reasonable approach to medical care and figure out how to apply them to their particular circumstances.

If we as a society reach a consensus on what constitutes a reasonable approach to medical care for elderly individuals in the final stages of their lives, then physicians will no longer need to burden patients and families with questions about the basic goals of treatment. Conversely, patients and families will not need to worry that physicians will make unilateral decisions based on their personal values. They will not need to fear undertreatment by a physician who believes that care should be drastically curtailed in all patients over 65 on economic grounds, or overtreatment by a physician who believes that life should be preserved at all costs. All elderly people will be assured of a single standard of care, depending on whether they are demented, robust, frail, or dying, with the detailed implementation of the general approach left to patient discretion.

Does such a model of medical decision making unfairly restrict individual choice? It is widely assumed that people have well-defined beliefs about what kind of care and how much care they want, beliefs readily deducible from their values and past actions. But in fact many such seemingly deeply ingrained beliefs, beliefs of the form "do everything to sustain my life" or "it is wrong to withhold food and fluids," evaporate in the face of a genuine understanding of what "doing everything" means or what feeding a comatose person through a gastrostomy tube is all about. The assumption that people's views follow directly from their religious beliefs and therefore that defining a set of acceptable goals would violate their religious freedom is equally flawed. It is widely held, for instance, that devout Catholics consistently espouse a single goal of care, the preservation of life, out of a moral conviction that they are obligated to accept all potentially life-sustaining interventions, however burdensome, and however unlikely they are to succeed. Papal decree says no such thing. There is in fact no requirement for Catholics to accede to what might be construed as extraordinary measures to prolong life.[17] Even more telling, in predominantly Catholic countries such as Ireland and Italy, there is no presumption in favor of life-extending treatment for the frail, the demented, or the dying elderly. Extremely ill old people are not routinely hospitalized. Instead, their families and physicians acknowledge that they are in the twilight of their lives, and provide supportive care in the home or, less often, in the nursing home.[18] What is at work in America is not so much the unfolding of deep-seated religious beliefs or community values[19] as the triumph of individualism, an individualism which holds that decisions about medical care are entirely a matter of individual preference, however misguided or confused that preference may be.[20]

If this framework for medical decision making in the elderly is reasonable, what are the obstacles to putting it into practice? First, there is the difficulty of defining who belongs in which category. Clearly I do not envisage and certainly would not endorse a bureaucratic system in which all elderly people underwent an evaluation, their status was determined, and they became card-carrying members of a particular group, with a specified benefits package accruing on the basis of their categorization. Moreover, the boundaries between the categories are blurred. Jennie Rosetti went from being robust to dying, but for a while it was not clear whether she was dying or merely very sick. As robust individuals gradually develop more impairments, they at some point become frail. Sometimes this frailty is due to an acute illness which leaves them with a new deficit (such as a stroke that causes paralysis) and sometimes it is due to a gradual process of deterioration, as with Grace Fitzgerald, whose arthritis progressively handicapped her. In the robust, the frail, or the demented, there is always the possibility that an acute illness will develop or a chronic illness become so severe that they enter the land of the dying. Some of the groups are not mutually exclusive: dementia can be combined with frailty or with dying. Finally, within the category of dementia, there are grades of severity. Maria Londino, when she first came to my office, was moderately demented. By the time she had been in the nursing home for a year and a half and was unable to walk independently, she was severely demented. The kind of medical care that made sense for Maria early in the course of her illness was not identical to the care that was appropriate later on.

The categories I have proposed are necessarily fluid—just as all the stages of life blend into one another. There is no hard and fast demarcation between infancy and childhood, or between childhood and adulthood. Adolescence arrives with a series of small explosions, not with a single bang. Old age creeps up on most of us: it is not determined by the possession of a Medicare card. And while there are perhaps some circumstances in which it is important to debate whether a person is a child or an adult, as for instance in thinking about whether a 13-year-old girl should unilaterally make the decision to undergo an abortion, for the most part we are aware of who is young and who is old, who is grown up and who is not. We have internalized the divisions, not merely on the basis of chronological age, but on the basis of physiological features and behavioral developments that accompany the stages of life. Similarly, we can identify as robust an elderly person who, despite chronic illness, is able to function with only a modicum of outside assistance. A frail elder is someone whose multiple medical problems render him or her vulnerable to the slightest physical upset, who cannot survive in the community without extensive help. And so forth, with dementia and with dying.

Once individuals are identified by their physicians as robust, frail, demented, or dying, they or their families need to be persuaded of the appropriateness of the kind of care outlined in this book, given their condition. Patients and prospective patients will, I hope, change their attitudes as they become exposed to the realities of being old and sick—personally, through friends, through stories like those told here, and above all through exposure to ways to treat patients without maximalist therapy.

Even if patients and their families accept my schema and if physicians are willing to endorse it, institutional changes will be necessary to make it possible to provide the kind of high-quality, non-procedure-oriented medical care that is entailed by this approach. The changes will need to come in the areas of nursing homes, hospitals, and health insurance. Most of these changes are beyond the reach of the individual; they are changes that will need to come from policymakers, legislators, and health care professionals. However, in each arena there are some changes that can take place through personal and collective efforts.

Nursing Homes

The nursing home is one institution that will have to change. It is no wonder that Grace Fitzgerald dreaded the prospect of entering a nursing home. And yet she was fortunate: she was so anxious alone at home, and so lonely, and so incapacitated, that entering a nursing home was a tremendous relief for her. The home she entered was of sufficiently high quality and the other residents on her floor were mentally intact enough that Grace could actually find a community in her new home. The majority of American nursing homes, however, are too small to be truly successful in separating those with high-level cognitive functioning from the demented, the quietly demented from the screamers, and the screamers from the wanderers. To be uprooted from one's home is traumatic enough; to be thrust into a new environment in which there is no one to converse with, or where the other residents invade one's already limited privacy or appear menacing in their behavior, must surely be devastating.

Grouping nursing home residents according to their level of impairment is just the first step in the direction of demedicalizing nursing home care. Gradually over the course of the century, and especially since the passage of Medicaid in 1965, nursing homes have evolved from comfortable old age homes to highly regulated medical care institutions. The old age home of the nineteenth and early twentieth century was established as a philanthropic undertaking by a religious or ethnic group to care for the working poor of their community. In the Boston area, for example, the Burnap Free Home for Aged Women was established in 1901 for elderly Protestant women; the German Ladies Aid Society of Boston was founded in 1893 for those of German descent; the Baptist Home in Cambridge was created in 1892 to support aged members.[21] By virtue of their admission requirements of community residency, usually of at least ten years' duration, these facilities served people who often already knew each other and had much in common. A typical candidate for the Winchester Home for Aged Women in the

Charlestown section of Boston, for instance, was a 74-year-old seamstress whose deceased husband had been a watchman in the Charlestown navy yard. At the time of her application for admission in 1909, she had lived in Charlestown for forty years and was certain to know a goodly number of the other wives of machinists, masons, and painters who inhabited the home.[22]

Since nineteenth-century old age homes were explicitly sectarian, they could provide the services of a minister of the appropriate denomination; since they were culturally homogeneous, they could guarantee that the residents would be served familiar kinds of food, that they would celebrate personally meaningful holidays, and that they would hear music that they knew and loved. Despite the loss of privacy resulting from living in an institution, despite the rules about coming down to breakfast every day or signing out before leaving, they could feel they were at home.

Contemporary nursing homes, by contrast, are overwhelmingly nonsectarian. They tend to be too large to have the intimacy of a home but too small to be able to group residents by their capacities: of the 19,100 nursing homes in the United States, 33 percent have fewer than 50 beds, but these homes account for only 9 percent of the total nursing home beds. The vast majority are over 50 beds but under 200, with 61 percent of the homes and 70 percent of the beds in this category. A mere 6 percent of all homes have over 200 beds, accounting for 20% of all beds.[23] The majority of homes are proprietary institutions, run for profit, with only a quarter either nonprofit or government-affiliated.

The typical nursing home is structured like a hospital rather than a true home, with long corridors of two-bed or even three- and four-bed rooms and a central nursing station. Every resident has a medical record; medications are dispensed by nurses; and doctors' orders determine whether residents can go to the bathroom on their own, if they may have alcohol on special occasions, and what they are given to eat, just as occurs in a hospital. The experience of living in a nursing home is also dramatically colored by government regulation affecting such facilities, regulations that are intended to ensure quality care but that often have the side effect of adversely affecting the quality of life.[24] Entering a nursing home, for most individuals, entails giving up their primary physician because regulations require that patients see their doctors in the facility rather than in the office, and most physicians are unwilling to see patients in the nursing home because of the inconvenience and a very low reimbursement rate. Regulations determine the frequency of physician visits, a rule meant to guarantee that patients are not neglected. In fact, by mandating that patients be seen every thirty days or every sixty days even in the absence of any acute problem, the rules promote perfunctory visits. Regulations also influence what medications patients receive, what laboratory tests are ordered, and the style of medical practice. In response to well-documented reports of overuse of medication, the Health Care Financing Administration has promulgated an algorithm for administering psychotropic medications which removes the need for physician discretion and judgment in prescribing. Although there has been little attempt to regulate laboratory tests directly, inspection teams reviewing nursing homes for recertification expect a certain frequency of laboratory tests, despite the absence of any good data justifying regular, frequent laboratory tests in the nursing home setting.

The structure of modern nursing homes, their size, their for-profit status, their nonsectarianism, and the government rules that regulate them are all conducive to the development of nursing homes as medical institutions rather than homes. It would be naive to believe that nursing homes can be remade in the image of the nineteenth-century old age home. Today's typical nursing home residents are older and need more help with activities of daily living than did their predecessors a century ago. But while they need more help in dressing, bathing, toileting, and eating, they are often not any sicker than their counterparts in the community. In fact, 90 percent of the care delivered in nursing homes is given by nurses' assistants or aides—the people who do the bathing, dressing, toileting, and feeding. Only 10 percent of the care is given by nurses or physical therapists, because while nursing home residents have more needs than could be met by an old-fashioned mom-and-pop establishment, they do not as a rule require more than episodic acute medical care. There is no intrinsic reason why they could not live in homes with their own personal possessions, and with recreational, educational, and other social programs that were oriented to their own background and interests.

The desirability of dramatically improving the quality of life in nursing homes is no mere do-gooder's dream. We can wish that we would all be in Nadine Chang's position as we age, with the family and the financial resources to remain at home, rather than in Grace Fitzgerald's situation, with one overburdened daughter and a very small bank account. The latest estimates are that 43 percent of individuals who turned 65 in 1990 will spend at least some time in a nursing home before death. About half of these will be short stays, designed for people who need rehabilitation or recuperation after an acute illness, or who literally enter the nursing home to die. The other half will be long stays, lasting at least one year.[25] The numbers of people who will spend time in a nursing home, most of whom will die in the home and many of whom will spend a good long time in the home, are surely large enough to stimulate far greater public interest in changing the nature of nursing homes.

It would be unrealistic to expect everyone to join a consumer lobbying group focused on promoting change in nursing homes. Ultimately, change will come from policymakers, from academics at universities and think tanks, from legislators, and from the long-term care industry itself. But there are at least two ways in which individuals, working within their own communities and households, can begin to make a difference. First, they can strongly encourage their church or synagogue or community center to build its own nursing home or life care community, intended for its members as they age. Such facilities would feature whatever ethnic foods, holiday celebrations, and linguistic requirements are appropriate to their group. Just as many organizations build their own nursery schools and parochial or other private schools, and subsidize their own low-income housing, as the population ages these same organizations need to think about supporting their aging members. There are already Armenian Homes, Swedish Homes, and Jewish Homes; there need to be many more such institutions, designed to the specifications of their future inhabitants.

Second, at a private level, individuals should begin purchasing long-term care insurance policies in ever-greater numbers. As the demand rises, the variety of policies will proliferate. Right now, private long-term care insurance pays for a negligible fraction of the expense of nursing home care. If there were an infusion of private funds into nursing homes, to bolster the paltry Medicaid income, this too might permit the expansion of programs in nursing homes. It might also allow for architectural changes such as the creation of more private rooms that would have a real effect on improving quality of life.

Hospitals

For the vast majority of patients, whether robust, frail, demented, or dying, home care is preferable to institutional care for treatment of acute illness if technically feasible. Older people tend to do better in a familiar environment. Even individuals who are normally mentally acute may become confused if they have a fever or are short of breath or are in pain. Being in an alien environment when your mind is not at its sharpest can have devastating consequences: you may have trouble locating the bathroom in the middle of the night; groping around in the semi-darkness, you are likely to trip and fall. The nurses, in a misguided attempt to encourage patients to use the call light to summon help if they need to get up during the night, will put up the metal siderails on both sides of the bed. As a result, older people on awakening and finding they need to go to the bathroom will discover to their astonishment that their bed has turned into some sort of a cage. Uncomprehending, and having no recollection of the previous day's conversation in which the nurse had exhorted them to call for help, knowing only that they need to get up, they will in desperation climb over the rails, this time falling from a greater height and fracturing a hip.

The physical unfamiliarity of the hospital—the unexpected side-rails, the absent night lights, and the displacement of familiar objects—is not the only disadvantage of institutionalization for medical treatment. The hospital is a total institution,[26] a highly structured environment run by administrators, doctors, and nurses, in which patients are expected to surrender control over their activities in exchange for competent and efficient medical treatment. The doctor decides what blood tests the patients should have, and technicians appear without warning to draw the blood. Similarly, the doctor orders X-rays, and orderlies appear with a stretcher or a wheelchair to whisk the patients off to the radiology suite, perhaps without their knowing in advance. With medication it is the same story: the nurse appears with a cupful of pills and stands over the patients while they dutifully down the prescribed potions. A new drug may have been discussed with them—certainly a medication known potentially to have major side effects, such as a chemotherapeutic agent against cancer, would have been discussed. But otherwise, when the medications are regarded as commonplace, it is one for the heart and one for the breathing and one to help you sleep, with little more by way of introduction or explanation. Diets are prescribed along with tests and medications. Patients usually have some choice of food and typically select items from a fairly lengthy menu. But the doctor decides whether the patients are to have a low-fat diet, or a diet with no added salt, or a diet without sweets, with the result that the physician has ultimate control over the quantity, and to a large degree, the taste of the food. The effect of the lack of control over tests, medications, and diet—not to mention over whether patients are allowed to get out of bed, walk down the hall, or go home—is often regression. Hospitalized patients in general, but especially older patients, quite rightly perceive that they are being treated like small children. Their typical response to the situation is to regress. They become docile and dependent, as befits their infantilized condition.[27]

The rigid structure of the hospital and the disorienting physical environment are both invitations to disaster for older patients. But even more insidious is the underlying philosophy of medical practice, which cannot readily be altered by simple maneuvers such as installing night lights and carpeting, putting beds closer to the floor, and allowing patients to "sign up" for diagnostic tests, thereby exercising some degree of control over their daily schedule. The guiding principles of medical practice are to be as certain as possible of the diagnosis, and then to employ whatever treatment is most likely to ensue in cure. Doctors in general are uncomfortable with the idea of treating with less than maximal certainty about the diagnosis, even when the test needed to marginally improve the probability of a given diagnosis carries with it a substantial cost.[28] The culture of the hospital also fosters the use of tests and procedures to confirm or exclude diagnoses. Simply having ready access to sophisticated X-ray machines and high-powered sub-specialists vastly increases the use of technology, often without any clear improvement in function and quality of life. In fact, studies comparing family physicians, internists, endocrinologists, and cardiologists have convincingly demonstrated that the major difference in their approach to treatment is a progressive increase in the number of tests ordered and the rate of hospitalization, even after adjusting for differences among their patients.[29] Comparing group practices that have laboratory facilities on site and those without demonstrates that the physicians with direct access to a laboratory order more tests.[30]

When older people get sick and enter a hospital, they are plunged into a new world, a world with an alien landscape, foreign laws and customs, and a dominant culture whose basic tenets are to test and to treat. For the robust elderly the trip is like any voyage abroad— tiring, a bit disorienting, but overall highly satisfying. For patients who are demented, the trip to the hospital may be frightening and overwhelming. Far from being a healing environment, the hospital may actually prove to impede recovery as test after test is inconclusive because of lack of patient cooperation and as the patients suffer multiple setbacks from the measures taken to calm them. For frail older individuals, the hospital may be therapeutic, but it is fraught with risks. Powerful drugs selected from the hospital physician's armamentarium may be too much for their weak kidneys; the routine admission blood tests and X-rays may reveal lesions that are best left alone but that, in the culture of the hospital, are liable to lead to endoscopy, biopsy, or surgery. And for dying patients, the hospital with its lights and its noise, its doctors and nurses bent on cure, is often antithetical to the goals of palliation and relief of suffering.

Even though the hospital is so inhospitable to a large proportion of older patients, many elderly individuals have no one to take care of them at home, or are too sick from their acute illness to be safely kept home. How can they be taken care of without resorting to the hospital? One proposed solution is the geriatric special care unit, a separate hospital ward devoted exclusively to the care of the older patient.[31] Such units are hardly the norm, and a number have been tried and failed; instead of serving the needs of acutely ill older patients who ultimately are expected to return home, they have become dumping grounds for elderly individuals who are unable to take care of themselves and are awaiting nursing home placement. The few examples that remain have not consistently demonstrated their superiority over conventional hospital care in any of the dimensions measured, such as minimization of the length of stay or preservation of the ability of patients to carry out activities of daily living.

While it seems plausible that special care units staffed by nurses, doctors, social workers, and physical therapists with expertise in geriatrics would be better places for older patients than standard hospital wards, it is not surprising to me that they have not been unequivocally successful. By virtue of their location within a hospital, inpatient geriatric wards have the same ready access to sub-specialists and tests as do all other hospital wards. Often the same interns and residents who rotate through the emergency room, the intensive care unit, and the medical service also spend time on the geriatrics unit. They bring with them the same striving for certainty and orientation toward cure that are demanded of them in the remainder of their clinical work. Exposure to an interdisciplinary team and lectures on topics in geriatric medicine, while undoubtedly beneficial, cannot possibly be expected to counteract significantly the powerful effects of the surrounding medical culture.

If older people cannot be taken care of in their homes when they become ill, whether because there is no one to care for them or because they are too sick to survive without virtually continuous professional surveillance, then the next best solution is to care for them in free-standing infirmaries. A number of health maintenance organizations (HMOs) have set up this kind of facility. Designed to give relatively simple care, as medicine goes, these infirmaries have the capacity to take straightforward X-rays (films of the chest or abdomen or bones which can be performed by a technician and do not involve the introduction of catheters or the injection of dye) and to provide treatment such as intravenous fluids and medications. The physicians still have their test-ordering, procedure-happy orientation, but when faced with a relative paucity of technology, they tend to rely heavily on their clinical skills and judgment. They still have the option to transfer patients from the infirmary to the general hospital if they deteriorate or if they are truly felt to require more monitoring, testing, or treatment than can be provided where they are. But remarkably few patients with pneumonia, kidney infections, mild congestive heart failure, or any of a number of common conditions for which patients are routinely hospitalized are in fact transferred to a more acute setting. Surprisingly, there is currently great geographic variability in whether such patients are hospitalized at all: in cities with vast numbers of hospital beds and a high rate of physicians per capita, individuals with these conditions are hospitalized to a much larger extent than in cities with fewer doctors and hospital beds.[32] When given access to more tests and more sub-specialists, physicians routinely avail themselves of these, with no measurable improvement in outcome for patients. The few studies that have looked at the consequences of a decrease in available resources have found that physicians accommodate to the change, again without any discernible impact on the welfare of patients.[33]

For those older people who live in nursing homes, the nursing home can establish its own on-site infirmary. In some instances, residents in nursing homes who become acutely ill can stay "home" because they can get the around-the-clock care. But the staffing ratios at the nursing home are often inadequate, especially at night, to tend to an acutely sick person. Physician backup on site may be unavailable, and good care may be impossible without access to certain basics such as chest X-rays and blood and urine tests. A solution used by a number of larger nursing homes is to set aside a section of the facility to serve as an acute care unit, very much like the infirmaries of the HMOs. More nurses are assigned per patient in the special unit—nurses with greater experience in handling intravenous lines or looking at electrocardiograms or listening to patients' lungs. Usually the nursing home contracts with an outside laboratory to obtain electrocardiograms, X-rays, and blood tests. The capacity to start intravenous lines for administration of fluid and medication, and to place nasogastric tubes either for suctioning out the stomach or for pumping in food, is arranged through the services of physicians, physician assistants, or nurse practitioners. From the point of view of the nursing home residents, the temporary transfer to a special unit disrupts their routine to some degree, but the changes are on the order of moving from the bedroom to the living room so as to be next to a bathroom and the kitchen instead of a flight of stairs away. From the point of view of the medical practitioners, the social expectation is that care will be provided within the confines of the nursing home. The temptation to order a confirmatory test or to use the newest antibiotic or to call in the specialist is reduced because these approaches are downright inconvenient and moreover are frowned upon by the surrounding medical culture.

The substitution of infirmary care—whether as part of a health maintenance organization, university health service, nursing home, or neighborhood health center—for hospital care is a fundamental structural change that individual patients are in no position to institute. However, such a change is clearly in the financial interest of any managed care system. If the HMO contracts with a hospital to provide care to its patients, no matter how attractive a rate the HMO is able to negotiate, it would undoubtedly be cheaper to provide infirmary-style care on its own premises. The HMO will not have to subsidize the hospital's purchase of new equipment or pay for a 24-hour intravenous team or support free care. Surely it can provide simple inpatient medical care for substantially less than the day rate of urban hospitals. The role of the individual in furthering the creation of more intermediate-level health care facilities is to demonstrate support for the idea, show willingness to accept care at the existing sites, and, in the increasingly competitive world of HMOs, preferentially select those plans that offer infirmary care.

Health Insurance Reform

Health maintenance organizations constitute just one means by which health care is delivered. As of 1986, 4.6 percent of the population over 65 were enrolled in HMOs.[34] The vast majority of older people get their medical care through the fee-for-service sector rather than through a prepaid health plan. This situation is likely to remain unchanged, even with national health care reforms that favor managed care, because the Medicare system is expected to remain relatively intact. Medicare Part A coverage is automatically available at age 65 to all American citizens who qualify for social security. This provides for 80 percent of hospital care, laboratory fees, and assorted other medical expenses (after a sizable deductible has been met). Coverage for physician services, outpatient hospital care, certain supplies, and a few miscellaneous services is available for a premium through the optional Medicare Part B. And since the two parts of Medicare combined leave 20 percent of the allowed medical costs unreimbursed, plus a significant deductible and other expenses such as medications which are not covered at all, about two-thirds of the elderly opt for a third medical insurance policy, the so-called medi-gap coverage.[35]

The Medicare system will need to change too—and in more ways than simply providing coverage for infirmary care—if elderly patients are to have the infrastructure necessary to realize their goals for medical care. The frail and the demented elderly desperately need better long-term care insurance coverage. By long-term care, I mean both home care (home health aides to provide personal care, homemakers to do housework, physical therapists to aid in rehabilitation, and visiting nurses to make house calls) and nursing home care. I am repeatedly astonished as successive polls disclose that the general public persists in believing, erroneously, that Medicare pays for nursing home care and for all necessary home care services.[36] The fact is that Medicare pays for only 2 percent of all nursing home costs because it does not cover what it regards as custodial or maintenance care. Medicaid, the joint federal-state program for the poor, pays for 42 percent of all nursing home care; the elderly pay 50 percent out of pocket; other government programs (principally the Veterans Administration, which cares for individuals with service-related disabilities) pay 4 percent; and the remainder is covered by miscellaneous sources, including private long-term care insurance.[37] Since the average cost nationwide for a year in a nursing home ranges from $20,000 to $45,000[38]—and a private room in a better home can come to $75,000 a year—the vast majority of people who enter a nursing home rapidly consume all their savings and must apply for Medicaid. (In Massachusetts,

63 percent of elderly individuals who live alone in the community and enter a nursing home qualify for Medicaid within three months, 83 percent by one year, and 91 percent within two years.)[39]

The problem with Medicare is not merely that it fails to pay for nursing homes. After all, if individuals exhaust their resources by paying for long-term care out of pocket, they become eligible for Medicaid, which then picks up the tab. The more fundamental problem is that embedded in the current system is a bias favoring institutional over home care. The Medicare program has little incentive to increase its home care benefits because it has a cheaper alternative: if it fails to provide sufficient care, the elderly may have no choice but to enter a nursing home, at which point they become Medicaid's responsibility.

The Medicare program presents significant obstacles to elderly patients' realizing their goals of care, quite apart from the issue of nursing home coverage. The major long-term care benefit that is provided by Medicare, coverage of home care services, is inadequate to the needs of many of the elderly. Although home care is the fastest-growing segment of the Medicare budget, currently accounting for 3.8 percent of Medicare expenditures, the types of services covered have remained unchanged since Medicare's inception.[40] The robust elderly need access to nursing care, physical therapy, and unskilled help after suffering a hip fracture or heart attack to avoid becoming frail. Medicare pays for a limited number of skilled nursing visits after discharge from a hospital but will no longer pay for services once patients are viewed as stable, even if they have not returned to their baseline status. The demented and the frail need both unskilled and professional help to remain at home when they become ill. The home is far more likely than the hospital to be conducive to the kind of less technologically intensive care that I suggest is consistent with the goals of treatment for these groups. Medicare does provide for nursing visits in the setting of an acute illness, but a half-hour visit several times a week is hardly adequate to maintain a frail older person at home. The dying should have the benefit of a hospice program in order to realize their goals for medical care. But while Medicare pays for hospice, this benefit is available only to people who have a full-time caretaker at home. In practice this means that many of those who are dying and would be eager to accept the palliative approach of hospice are ineligible simply because they live alone.[41] If hospice is to work for individuals who do not have a spouse or privately paid help to care for them, it will need to supply personal care attendants. People who are dying are almost invariably too weak to care for themselves in the final days or weeks of their illness. At a minimum, they need help with bathing and dressing, cooking and cleaning.

Proposals abound for establishing a new long-term care system.[42] Many recommend a single, comprehensive system with only one payer. The most sweeping proposal would cover all medical and social services under a single public plan, including nursing, physical therapy, hospice, and homemaking, as well as nursing home care.[43] Various funding sources have been suggested, ranging from new taxes to private insurance to use of reverse mortgages. Expansion of Medicare to create a Part C for long-term care is one suggestion; the creation of a whole new program to supplant not only Medicare but the eighty or so other federal programs that devote some resources to the elderly is another approach.

As with nursing home reform, the general public will probably not be intimately involved with the details of any changes. Addressing the needs of the 37 million Americans who are uninsured is so pressing, as is controlling the rising cost of medical care, that most of the effort devoted to health care reform is centered on these problems. Precisely because that task alone is so monumental, the natural tendency is to ignore long-term care. But the public can play a very definite role in guaranteeing that there is a thorough restructuring of the long-term care system. Public views on health care have been a major factor in determining the outcome of both state and national elections. Polls and letters to congressmen have been shown to influence legislators at least as much as reports from academic think-tanks.[44] Without consistent, relentless public pressure, the temptation will be to postpone long-term care reform.

In addition to changes in institutional care and medical insurance, the behavior of physicians needs to change. Physicians tend not to talk to patients about the future and what it might hold for them; when physicians and patients do discuss preferences for future care, the doctors do not always abide by their patients' wishes; and whether or not physicians discuss plans with their patients, they tend to feel uncomfortable limiting care.

Physicians

The embarrassing fact is that physicians seldom broach the issue of life-sustaining treatments with patients, let alone engage in more far-reaching discussions about what lies in store for them and the possible goals of medical care. Multiple studies confirm that patients wish to discuss "what if," but physicians seldom raise the subject. One poll of 152 patients followed in a general medical clinic disclosed that although 68 percent wanted to discuss the use of life-sustaining treatment in the event of major illness, only 6 percent had in fact held such discussions.[45] Another study, focusing exclusively on individuals over 65, found that all 72 patients interviewed about their views felt comfortable discussing such matters, but only one had previously had such a discussion with his physician.[46] The Patient Self-Determination Act (PSDA), which went into effect in 1991, is a legislative attempt to require that the subject of advance directives be raised, at least on admission to a hospital or nursing home. However, hospitals are already incorporating the obligation to inquire about living wills into the job of the admissions officer. Along with listing the address, social security number, health insurance information, and next of kin, hospital clerks are routinely asking patients whether they have a living will or whether they want one, and responding by checking off a box or handing out a pamphlet.[47] It seems clear that whatever the virtues of the PSDA, generating serious dialogue between doctors and patients about the realities of aging, dementia, and dying is not one of them.

Moreover, there is mounting evidence that in those cases where advance directives have been drawn up, physicians do not uniformly heed their instructions. In one of the most meticulously performed studies, 126 nursing home residents who had executed advance directives were followed prospectively for two years. Of these, 96 were hospitalized or died during the two years, but in only 75 percent of cases was the care given consistent with clearly expressed prior wishes.[48] Some of the lack of concordance was due to logistical problems: the living wills did not successfully travel with patients from the nursing home to the hospital. Another reason why patients' wishes were ignored was the conviction on the part of physicians that the advance directive did not really apply to the situation at hand. The patient might, for example, have said she did not want to be intubated for respiratory failure, but the physician might correctly understand that the patient really meant that she did not want to remain on a respirator for the rest of her life. If the machine was merely intended for temporary support during a treatable bout of pneumonia, the patient would find it eminently acceptable. The problem, in short, is with the nature of advance directives.

Some of the violations of patient preferences probably reflect physicians' reluctance to limit care. An analysis of just how far physicians are willing to go in limiting care ascertained that physicians have significant reservations about the kinds of requests made by competent, terminally ill patients that they are willing to honor. While fully 98 percent of those polled said they would honor a request to withhold intubation, only 86 percent stated that they would give high doses of narcotic medication for pain control if this might provoke respiratory depression and death, and only 59 percent agreed in theory to turn off a respirator if asked to do so by a patient.[49]

Physicians tend to feel uncomfortable limiting care—and not just because they suspect the patient did not truly want care limited or because they worry that their actions might directly kill their patients. Physicians are apprehensive about providing less than maximally intensive care because virtually all of medical training preaches the reverse. Medical school and residency training both stress making a diagnosis with as much certainty as possible, and then treating with whatever therapy has the greatest statistical chance of success, with little consideration of the effects of treatment on quality of life. Studies in medical journals further promote this attitude; they typically compare new drugs to old drugs (or to a placebo) and new operations to old techniques in terms of readily measurable outcomes such as mortality or numbers of strokes or heart attacks. Incorporating quality of life into the assessment of the relative merits of two approaches is just beginning to be used.[50]

The legal climate also conspires to deter physicians from limiting treatment. Doctors are afraid that they will be sued for having failed to institute the most aggressive therapy available. After all, patients may not have wanted any part of such treatment, but if the patient dies, he is not available to testify. Family members, whose views may have differed dramatically from those of the patient, are the ones left to sue. And although there have now been several successful suits for unwanted treatment, the majority of lawsuits continue to be for what is perceived as undertreatment. Finally, even though physicians are usually in a good position to defend themselves successfully in court if they treat in accordance with a patient's wishes, their goal is not only to win any possible lawsuit, but also to avoid altogether the arduous and painful process of being sued. Legal counsel rendered by hospital lawyers is often similarly biased in the direction of avoiding litigation, not merely ensuring that if there is a suit, the hospital and physician are likely to win.

Physicians are also inhibited by regulatory authorities from restricting medical care. In an attempt both to control costs and to assure quality of care, physicians are increasingly expected to practice medicine in accordance with fixed protocols.[51] The goal of protecting patients from unnecessary procedures is laudable. Studies based on indications for procedures established by panels of experts have found that as many as two-thirds of endarterectomies, one-fourth of coronary angiograms, and one-fourth of endoscopies are unwarranted.[52]

Unfortunately, setting standards for when a procedure might be reasonable tends to determine when it must be done. Instead of merely guaranteeing that interventions will not take place when they should not, the creation of criteria also implies that the interventions should take place whenever the criteria are met. There is no allowance for the possibility that empirical treatment of gastrointestinal bleeding with medications might be a reasonable approach in a frail 85-year-old. A physician might reason that a patient who is throwing up blood most likely has either an ulcer, gastritis (an irritation of the lining of the stomach that is not quite deep enough to qualify as an ulcer), or a tumor. Both of the first two disorders are often treated with medication that blocks acid formation in the stomach, thereby promoting healing. A gastric tumor, usually malignant, is rarely treatable and even more rarely curable. An elderly individual with multiple other medical problems would very likely not be an operative candidate. Thus the prime advantage of definitively establishing a diagnosis—of looking down into the stomach with an endoscope and obtaining a biopsy of the abnormal tissue—would be for purposes of prognosis, for knowing what to expect in the future. Similarly, demented elderly patients might meet all the formal criteria for undergoing cardiac catheterization, but their family might concur that given their overall level of function, their inability to understand and therefore to cooperate with an invasive procedure, and the possibility of controlling their anginal symptoms reasonably well with medications, they should not have the test. However, state professional review organizations, in accordance with their federal mandate, are increasingly critical of idiosyncratic decision making and are likely to censure a physician for prematurely discharging a patient who was hospitalized for angina and then sent home without an ostensibly indicated angiogram.[53] Although the physician could appeal the citation, probably successfully, on the grounds that the family declined the test, the simplest strategy would decidedly be to go ahead and schedule the procedure.

Patients and Families

The final barrier to instituting my approach to the medical care of elderly patients is patients and families themselves. My proposal, after all, calls for a lesser intensity of care for elderly people who are frail, demented, or dying. Despite the widespread concern that physicians inappropriately prolong the life of the dying, many patients and their relatives are profoundly ambivalent about what they perceive as limitations of care. With all the discussion of the high cost of care in the final year of life—the fraction of all Medicare expenditures used for care in the last year of life has remained stable at 28 percent from 1975 to 1988[54]—families are rightly suspicious that limitations in care may be motivated by a desire to save money. The commonly used phraseology of withdrawing, withholding, limiting, or abating care conveys the impression that something valuable is deliberately being denied to patients. When the matter is put this way, individuals are appropriately skeptical. The plight of Maria Londino, compelled to die in the coronary care unit, or Sam Schaeffer, who suffered repeated complications after his valve replacement, should highlight the fact that limiting care does not constitute deprivation. Rather, what is meant is the substitution of labor-intensive for capital-intensive care, the replacement of treatment focused on cure and life-prolongation by care whose aim is to maximize function.

Although patients are doubtful about whether physicians in particular or the health care system in general should make decisions to limit care, they are nonetheless eager to discuss their personal preferences. But study after study has found that patients want to talk about advance directives but have difficulty initiating the discussion with their primary physicians. The conclusion usually drawn by the authors of such studies is that physicians need to learn to bring up the topic of advance care planning.[55] Legislative requirements and a gradual process of education will probably ultimately change physicians' practices, but to facilitate and accelerate the change, patients should share the responsibility of bringing up the subject of future directions in care. Just as it is patients who need to come out and state that they are in the office because of double vision or burning on urination, it can be the patients who say they wish to discuss what to anticipate in the next few years.

Changes in hospitals, nursing homes, insurance coverage, and physicians' behavior would help lay the groundwork for a new approach to medical decision making in the elderly. Physicians need to define goals of care based on the overall condition of the individual; society as a whole needs to endorse this approach and then, within the boundaries determined by those goals, promote individual choice. But without the institutional framework needed to implement decisions arrived at in this way, the approach will founder. It is patients and their families who need to become advocates for change. Unless the twenty-five million elderly and their roughly fifty million children favor substituting infirmary care for hospital care, want to revamp nursing homes to make them more like homes and less like institutions, and vote for major modifications in long-term care insurance coverage, little will change. And if little changes, then older people will have difficulty implementing their preferences for care in the final years of their lives, however clear and well-thought-out their wishes, and however consonant their desires with the recommendations of their physicians.

❖ *Epilogue* ❖

My portraits of patients are snapshots, taken at a particular point in time: Nadine Chang, sitting in front of her television set, with a swollen leg; Claire Renan, eager to get her life over and done with when she learned she had rectal cancer. I have tried to provide a few images from earlier times, before the acute illness, to help create a fuller picture of each patient, to help situate each individual in the context of his or her life prior to becoming old and sick. I have tried to relate something about the person and not merely the technical facts of the case in order to underscore that the decisions regarding the kind of care to give cannot be based solely on abstract philosophical principles, but rather on a consideration of what the various possible strategies would involve for that person.

But I do not mean to suggest that the choices made in every individual case were or should have been entirely a reflection of the idiosyncratic preferences or beliefs of patients and their families. On the contrary, I believe that at the major branch-points along the decision tree—how aggressively to treat, whether to aspire to cure or to palliation—the general approach should be determined by the individual's overall condition: robust, frail, demented, or dying. More specific implementation of the general care plan is what should be determined by the individual's values, wishes, and personal circumstances. My argument is that almost everyone in

Richard Brown's predicament—bedridden, unable to speak or understand, incapable of experiencing joy or remorse—would not want invasive technology to prolong his existence, particularly when the technology itself would induce pain, fear, and bewilderment. Almost everyone in Panos Pappadokoulos's situation—vigorous and active at 85—if found to have complete heart block with a significant risk of fainting or sudden death, would opt for a pacemaker. Similarly, most people in Carol Richards's shoes, suffering from end-stage emphysema, would favor supportive care. Few people who truly acknowledge that there is no cure for their illness and that their death is imminent would want painful or at least highly unpleasant treatment, just for the sake of doing something. And most people, if they knew that only a respirator could sustain them and if they understood that respirator-dependence meant indefinite attachment to a bulky machine that would prevent them from talking and eating and leaving the hospital, would regard such an intervention as torment rather than treatment. Finally, most people who understand what it means to be frail, what is entailed by open heart surgery for a man like Sam Schaeffer, whose vital organs were operating on only one cylinder, would opt for a less aggressive approach to treatment. They would favor a course that offers more than palliation but probably less than cure.

How the approach I propose would play out in real life, and how it would differ from the way medicine is usually practiced today, is best seen using a video camera. We need to start filming when our subject is well, and travel forward through time to glimpse the decision-making process in action.

———————

Once Ginger Johnson had her third and last child at age 36, she assiduously avoided doctors. Shortly after her sixtieth birthday, she grudgingly allowed her daughter Meredith to take her to a community health fair, where she learned that her blood pressure was sky-high, her cholesterol was quite high, and her blood sugar was a little high. Ginger felt perfectly well and was extremely reluctant to see a doctor because she was certain she would be handed one or more prescriptions for medication. From her point of view, all medications were poisons.

When I saw Ginger in the office, her fears were confirmed. I checked her blood pressure multiple times, and it was always elevated. I repeated her blood sugar measurement, this time on an empty stomach, and it was still too high. I ordered a full lipid profile, which disclosed that Ginger had far too much LDL, the "bad" cholesterol, and not nearly enough HDL, the "good" cholesterol. We agreed that she would go on a low-fat, low-salt diet and avoid sweets. She would take advantage of the mild fall weather and take a brisk walk several times a week.

After six weeks, Ginger came back and reported that she was sick and tired of eating fish and chicken. She had lost only one pound despite not having touched a single dessert. The weather had changed markedly: Boston had already had its first snow, and she could not possibly continue her exercise regimen. To make matters worse, despite all her efforts, her blood pressure, sugar, and cholesterol were still up. I discussed the risk of a stroke or a heart attack in light of her consistently high blood pressure, and she reluctantly agreed to a trial of medication. We decided to hold off on cholesterol-lowering medication so as to give diet a bit more of a chance. Her diabetes was mild enough that she did not yet unequivocally warrant medication.

Fortunately, the antihypertensive medication agreed with Ginger. She bought a cookbook that helped liven up the chicken and fish dishes. Her sugars remained borderline, and her cholesterol fell to a more acceptable range.

For five years Ginger did very well. She continued to work as a salesperson in a local department store on a part-time basis and spent much of the remaining time babysitting for her five grandchildren. She was active in a garden club, proudly showing off photographs of her floral arrangements and prizes she won for her work. She led a full and varied life. She was, as she put it, as content as an overweight widow who was graduating from middle age could expect to be. Ginger had even become reconciled both to the pill she took daily to control her blood pressure and to her biannual visits to see me.

Shortly after her sixty-fifth birthday, Ginger came in for a regularly scheduled appointment. I performed a physical examination, did blood tests and an electrocardiogram, and we talked. Ginger felt as well as when we had first met—perhaps, she confessed, even a little better now that she had succeeded in losing a few pounds. I assured her that she in fact was in good condition. She had several medical problems that needed monitoring, but nothing that should interfere with her life. I indicated that while the social security administration felt she had reached a major milestone, I did not think she had crossed any magic threshold. My approach to her medical care, if she developed any new problems, would remain what it had always been.

At age 70, without any warning, Ginger Johnson developed crushing chest pain associated with profuse sweating, dry heaves, and difficulty in breathing. I sent her directly to the hospital emergency room, where an electrocardiogram proved she was having a heart attack. She was admitted to the coronary care unit and, after a rocky day or two, did well. She did so well that in a week, she wanted to be discharged. I had to argue with her to remain in the hospital for further testing in order to determine if she was at risk for subsequent heart damage. She was extremely skeptical, but after ten years as my patient she knew me well enough to recognize that my style of practice was cautious and conservative. Moreover, I had long ago given up trying to persuade her to do anything health-related that was of only marginal benefit. She trusted me enough to appreciate that I did not push for intervention unless I thought it was extremely important. Ginger gave in. I was tremendously relieved, especially when the pictures from the catheterization showed impressive constrictions in each of three coronary arteries.

She underwent uncomplicated bypass surgery and remained free of further heart trouble, able to maintain her active schedule.

Ginger did not, however, live happily ever after. A year after her open heart surgery, she came to me frantic because she had discovered a lump in her breast. I tried to be optimistic, reminding her that not all lumps were cancerous. That was true, of course, but in a 71-year-old woman most lumps *are* cancerous. Her mammogram showed the streaks of calcium typical of breast cancer, and a biopsy eliminated whatever small doubt remained. I was still guardedly optimistic. Breast cancer may be slow-growing in older women, and Ginger had no evidence to suggest any spread of the tumor. She consented to a mastectomy and then treatment with tamoxifen, an anti-estrogen that is often extremely successful in keeping breast cancer at bay.

Again Ginger did well. She had slowed down a little: she became tired easily and decided to retire from her part-time job. She was glad her grandchildren had outgrown the need for babysitters, though she regretted that they and their parents were all moving away. Her blood sugar, which had always been on the high side, could no longer be controlled by diet. Her blood pressure, too, had begun creeping up. Instead of the one pill a day she had agreed to many years earlier, she now took three different medications for her blood pressure and another one for diabetes. She was developing cataracts in both eyes, as well as other eye problems stemming from the diabetes. Despite these failings, I told Ginger on the occasion of her 72-year-old checkup, I still regarded her as robust. Her blood pressure and diabetes, after all, were well regulated, though a substantial amount of medication was needed to achieve that feat. Her breast cancer was cured or at least dormant. Her diminished energy level notwithstanding, she did her own housekeeping and led an active social life.

A mere six months later, Ginger's world began to crumble. She slipped on the bathroom floor, perhaps because her vision in the dark was no longer as acute as it had been, fracturing her hip. She smiled at me mournfully as I checked her electrocardiogram and blood pressure in anticipation of surgery. "It's been an operation every year, three years running. I wonder what the next operation will be?" We joked that maybe one of the cataracts would be ready to come out after all. There was always her gallbladder and her appendix, I reminded her.

The surgery went smoothly, but Ginger never recovered her former spunk. She was fortunate enough to be accepted by a rehabilitation hospital for extensive physical therapy, unlike the 60 percent of individuals who break their hips and as a result enter a nursing home.[1] At the end of two weeks, Ginger was able to walk using a cane. But she found that she had difficulty negotiating the half-dozen stairs leading to her house. She also had difficulty reaching down to put on her stockings or tie her shoes. And without her cane, she felt too unsteady to be able to use both hands to cook or clean. The net effect was that Ginger, who had always been totally independent, now needed someone to cook for her, to shop for her, to clean her house, and even to help dress her. Until she installed a ramp leading to the house, she was also a prisoner in her own home. Grudgingly, Ginger accepted the need for personal help. She hired a young woman to come in for four hours every morning, an arrangement she agreed to only because she expected it to be temporary.

It was not temporary. Despite additional physical therapy at home, Ginger remained dependent on her cane. Just when she seemed to be making some progress, she fell again. This time her confidence was shattered, though her bones fortunately were not. She did not trust herself anymore and began requiring more help, not less.

Ginger's world shrank down to her house and an occasional outing with her children, none of whom lived locally but all of whom came to visit as often as their busy schedules allowed. She had one close friend who came to play cards with her. She could no longer tend her garden but fussed over the houseplants which adorned every window sill. The light bothered her eyes, making it difficult for her to read. She watched television and took a great many catnaps. And then she began having difficulty breathing.

My first thought was that her shortness of breath was due to a failing heart. A chest X-ray proved otherwise. Half of Ginger's left lung was filled with fluid. I knew all too well that probably meant her breast cancer, quiescent for two years, had metastasized. A small needle inserted above a rib in her back to withdraw a sample of the fluid confirmed that yes, the breast cancer was back.

Ginger was very discouraged. She was ready to give up. I urged her to put up with a bone scan to determine whether there were other metastases. It was important, I felt, to assess the situation fully, to evaluate the magnitude of the problem, in order to figure out what treatment might be beneficial. After a good deal of procrastination, Ginger agreed. She was lucky: the only discernible metastases at that point were to her lung. I pointed out that many people with metastatic breast cancer live for years with their disease. Chemotherapy, while seldom curative, has the potential to cause regression of the cancer and to prevent further spread. She was no longer the vigorous woman she had been at the time of her bypass surgery, but neither was she terminally ill. She might still have a few good years left.

The oncologist to whom I sent Ginger agreed that she would most likely benefit from treatment. He recommended a cocktail of three different drugs, most of which she could take by mouth. She would need to have her blood counts monitored carefully, since the major side effect of the medication was to depress the functioning of the bone marrow; she would be at risk of serious infections if her counts became too low. The oncologist also recommended a wig, since one of the medications would make her lose all her hair. Again, Ginger went along.

For a year, the chemotherapy worked. The fluid in her lung subsided. Apart from the inconvenience of visits to the doctor and the frequent blood tests, apart from the shock of actually seeing herself go bald, she was fine. Her three children and her five grandchildren put together a magnificent party for Ginger's seventy-fifth birthday. She basked in their affection; she reveled in her role as matriarch; and her family marveled that she barely touched the food.

Ginger did not touch the food because she had been losing her appetite. For the first time in fifteen years, she had lost a significant amount of weight. She was so pleased that she did not admit to herself that something was wrong until she noticed her skin had a yellow tinge. She arrived at my office for an urgent appointment and joked that maybe my prediction from long ago had come true: maybe she had gallstones. We smiled, but we both knew she did not have gallstones. She had metastases to the liver from her breast cancer.

By the time she saw her oncologist a week later, she also had aches and pains in her back. The cancer was on a rampage, having spread both to her liver and to her bones. The fluid in her lung had returned as well, and there was a hint of fluid in the other lung. Clearly the chemotherapy was no longer working. Ginger's oncologist suggested another round of chemotherapy, with a different concoction of drugs. She shook her head and said she needed to think it over.

Ginger came back to see me one more time. She came with her oldest daughter, Meredith, the daughter who had dragged her to the health fair fifteen years earlier and had insisted that she see a doctor for her blood pressure and her high cholesterol. We talked, first about the facts, then about the options, finally about what we each thought. It was difficult for me to be blunt as I looked at Ginger, still plump despite her weight loss, the whites of her eyes now bright yellow, her lemon-complexioned face crowned by a shock of thick brown hair. (If she was going to wear a wig, she had decided, she might as well seize the opportunity to be rid of her gray hair.) I groped for the right words and finally simply said that she had very little time left and that chemotherapy was more likely to ruin what time she had than to prolong it.

Meredith began to cry, and Ginger herself got a bit choked up. Her voice sounded thin, high-pitched, weak. But what she said was very clear. She did not want any more chemotherapy. In fact, she wanted nothing further to do with hospitals, needles, or X-rays. Her daughter had a guest room. She would pack up her most precious possessions, move to her daughter's house, and stay there until she died.

Ginger and her daughter left the office and went home to pack. I got on the telephone to make the necessary arrangements. Lining up services by long distance was complicated, but feasible. Meredith's doctor accepted Ginger as a patient and made a hospice referral. Ginger drew on her dwindling savings to pay for 24-hour care by a nurse's aide. She died two weeks later.

Death and loss are always sad. But Ginger had had a rich life. As long as she had been robust, she had received and benefited from all that medical technology had to offer: she had had bypass surgery, she had had a total hip replacement and a mastectomy, and she had been given the most sophisticated treatment available to control her high blood pressure, her diabetes, and her high cholesterol. When, after her hip surgery, she became frail, she continued to profit from medical treatment, to the extent warranted by her weakened state. She had a thoracentesis to remove fluid from her lung; she had a bone scan; and she received chemotherapy, a kind that was chosen for its relatively mild side effects. And once she moved from being frail—from having heart disease and an artificial hip, diabetes, and breast cancer, with resultant reduction in her mobility, her ability to care for herself, and her enjoyment of life—to being terminally ill, she also received high-quality medical care. She was kept comfortable with modern pain-control techniques and intensive personal care until the very end. At each of the last stages of her life, Ginger and I reviewed her status, reevaluated the goals of care, and made subsequent treatment decisions based on those discussions.

The truth about Ginger Johnson is quite different from the idealized picture I have presented. She did have high blood pressure, diabetes, and high cholesterol. She did have a heart attack. But there the divergence between fantasy and reality begins. When Ginger had her heart attack, the cardiologist told her she was too old to consider bypass surgery. I overheard him comment to another physician that he had read all those studies about too much money being spent on old people, and he for one was not going to contribute to that travesty.[2] I pleaded that she was physiologically and functionally youthful and urged her to seek a second opinion. Ginger, never one to be eager to have things done to her, was satisfied that if the expert thought she should be treated with medication, that was fine with her.

She was one of the lucky ones who did not have a second heart attack—perhaps she did not have a chance because the breast cancer got her first. She did have severe angina, disabling chest pain, every few days. Her pain was so frightening that she began avoiding any activity involving the slightest exertion for fear it would trigger the pain.

In actual fact, Ginger Johnson was forced to change her insurance coverage after she quit her job as a salesperson. The new health plan she joined drastically limited her choice of physicians. I was no longer able to be her doctor. When her breast cancer recurred, she was referred to an oncologist who was adamant that Ginger undergo aggressive chemotherapy. He started her on a protocol which made her throw up in addition to losing her hair. With each cycle of treatment, her blood counts dipped into the danger range. She had three hospitalizations within six months for fever in the setting of a very low white blood cell count, and each time she was put on reverse precautions—everyone entering her room had to wear a surgical gown, mask, and gloves to prevent spreading germs to her—while she got multiple intravenous antibiotics. When fluid developed in her lung, the oncologist told her that the best way to treat her was to take her to the operating room and remove the lining surrounding the lung so that fluid would no longer be able to accumulate. When, despite the chemotherapy, bone metastases popped up, the oncologist sent Ginger for a course of radiation treatments to the bone and prescribed a new chemotherapy regimen. Ginger died in the hospital, alone, with intravenous lines in both arms through which her well-intentioned doctors poured huge quantities of blood, antibiotics, and nutrients in their relentless fight against death.

With some degree of preventive medicine and a good deal of luck, we will all live to a ripe old age. A small minority will remain vigorous until the very end and then suddenly expire. The vast majority will go through a phase of frailty, and some will pass through a period of dementia, before entering the realm of the dying. Only if patients, potential patients, families, and physicians acknowledge that what is right for the robust is not the same as that which is right for the frail, the demented, and the dying, and only if physicians tell patients where they stand, can we hope that our final years will more closely resemble my fantasy about Ginger than the reality.

But it is not enough for individual physicians to delineate reasonable goals of medical care for individual elderly patients, based on their functional status. Ideally, we will achieve a societal consensus about what constitutes a standard approach to care. Once there is agreement about the aims of medicine in an aging population, we can modify Medicare reimbursement for medical interventions accordingly. If the explicit goals of care for the demented and the dying, for example, are incompatible with hospitalization in an intensive care unit, then Medicare should not be expected to pay for such treatment. If the agreed-upon goal of care for the robust is cure, then Medicare should cover curative cancer surgery. If the goal of care for the frail is maximization of function, then Medicare should not be expected to pay for procedures that are far more likely to induce further disability than to produce benefit.[3]

The savings generated by such a policy could be used to develop the new medical institutions needed to permit implementation of the goals of care, institutions such as infirmaries and radically restructured nursing homes.

Without institutional change, the realization of a just, rational, and decent approach to illness near the end of life will be difficult. Without change, both in institutions and in the framework for decision making, older people and their families will be unprepared for the illnesses they are destined to develop as they age, ill-equipped to handle the decisions about treatment of those illnesses that will be foisted upon them. They will risk being subjected to excessive technological intervention or, at the other extreme, be denied scientifically validated medical treatment on the grounds of age alone. The path to change begins with a shared understanding of the experience of being old and sick, an understanding we can arrive at through journeys to the world of Richard Brown, Rebecca Landsman, Claire Renan, Sam Schaeffer, and their fellow-sufferers in the twilight of life.

Notes ❖ *Index*

❖ *Notes* ❖

Prologue

1. E. Schneider and J. Guralnik, "The Aging of America: Impact on Health Care Costs," *Journal of the American Medical Association* 263 (1990): 2335–2340.
2. D. Evans, H. Funkenstein, M. Albert, et al., "Prevalence of Alzheimer's Disease in a Community Population of Older Persons," *Journal of the American Medical Association* 262 (1989): 2551–2556.
3. U.S. Senate Special Committee on Aging, *Aging America: Trends and Projections* (Washington, D.C.: U.S. DHHS, 1988), Table 4-8, p. 114.
4. National Center for Health Statistics, Monthly Vital Statistics Report, April 1990.
5. U.S. Senate Special Committee on Aging, *Aging America*, p. 12.
6. Ibid., pp. 125–126.
7. Schneider and Guralnik, "The Aging of America."
8. T. McKeown, *The Role of Medicine: Dream, Mirage, or Nemesis?* (Princeton, N.J.: Princeton University Press, 1979).
9. L. Verbrugge, "Longer Life but Worsening Health: Trends in Health and Mortality of Middle-aged and Older Persons," *Milbank Memorial Fund Quarterly* 62 (1984): 475–519.
10. S. Abramowitz, "Pain, as a Matter of Policy," *New York Times*, October 24, 1989, p. 27.
11. C. Kjellstrand, "Who Should Decide about Your Death?" *Journal of the American Medical Association* 267 (1992): 103–104.
12. H. Aaron and W. Schwartz, *The Painful Prescription: Rationing Hospital Care* (Washington, D.C.: The Brookings Institution, 1984); V. Fuchs,

"Though Much Is Taken: Reflections on Aging, Health, and Medical Care," *Milbank Memorial Fund Quarterly* 62 (1984): 43–66.

13. D. Blumenthal, M. Schlesinger, J. Drumheller, et al., "The Future of Medicare," *New England Journal of Medicine* 314 (1986): 722–728; K. Davis, "Aging and the Health Care System: Economic and Structural Issues," *Daedalus* 115 (1986): 227–246.

14. D. Callahan, *Setting Limits: Medical Goals in an Aging Society* (New York: Simon and Schuster, 1987); N. Daniels, *Just Health Care* (Cambridge: Cambridge University Press, 1985).

15. T. Beauchamp and J. Childress, *Principles of Biomedical Ethics* (New York: Oxford University Press, 1989).

1. Robbed of Mind and Memory

1. R. Katzman, "Alzheimer's Disease," *New England Journal of Medicine* 314 (1986): 964–973.

2. R. Terry and R. Katzman, "Senile Dementia of the Alzheimer's Type," *Annals of Neurology* 14 (1983): 497–506.

3. D. Evans, H. Funkenstein, M. Albert, et al. "Prevalence of Alzheimer's Disease in a Community Population of Older Persons," *Journal of the American Medical Association* 262 (1989): 2551–2556.

4. E. Hing, "Use of Nursing Homes by the Elderly: Preliminary Data from the National Nursing Home Survey," Advance Data No. 135, National Center for Health Statistics, May 14, 1987.

5. D. Hilfiker, "Allowing the Debilitated to Die," *New England Journal of Medicine* 308 (1983): 716–719.

6. T. Beauchamp and J. Childress, *Principles of Biomedical Ethics,* 3rd ed. (New York: Oxford University Press, 1989).

7. B. Mishkin, *A Matter of Choice: Planning Ahead for Health Care Decisions* (Washington, D.C.: American Association of Retired Persons, 1986), pp. 42–44.

8. T. Hill and D. Shirley (Choice in Dying), *A Good Death: Taking More Control at the End of Your Life* (Reading, Mass.: Addison-Wesley, 1992), pp. 145–147.

9. L. Emanuel and E. Emanuel, "The Medical Directive: A New Comprehensive Advance Care Document," *Journal of the American Medical Association* 261 (1989): 3288–3293.

10. D. Oken, "What to Tell Cancer Patients: A Study of Medical Attitudes," *Journal of the American Medical Association* 175 (1961): 1120–1128.

11. D. Novack, R. Plumer, R. Smith, et al., "Changes in Physicians' Attitudes

toward Telling the Cancer Patient," *Journal of the American Medical Association* 241 (1979): 897–900.

12. M. Drickamer and M. Lachs, "Should Patients with Alzheimer's Disease Be Told Their Diagnosis?" *New England Journal of Medicine* 326 (1992): 947–951.

13. D. Orentlicher, "Advance Medical Directives," *Journal of the American Medical Association* 263 (1990): 2365–2367.

14. J. Menikoff, G. Sachs, and M. Siegler, "Beyond Advance Directives: Health Care Surrogate Laws," *New England Journal of Medicine* 327 (1992): 1165–1169.

15. E. Brody, "The Informal Support System and Health of the Future Aged," in C. Gaitz, G. Niedereh, and N. Wilson, eds., *Aging 2000: Our Health Care Destiny* (New York: Springer Verlag, 1985), pp. 174–189.

16. P. Greco, K. Schulman, and R. Lavizzo-Mourey, "The Patient Self-Determination Act and the Future of Advance Directives," *Annals of Internal Medicine* 115 (1991): 639–643.

17. D. Murphy, A. Murray, B. Robinson, and E. Campion, "Outcomes of Cardiopulmonary Resuscitation in the Elderly," *Annals of Internal Medicine* 111 (1989): 199–205.

18. R. Veatch, *Death, Dying, and the Biological Revolution* (New Haven: Yale University Press, 1989), p. 78.

19. N. Brown and D. Thompson, "Nontreatment of Fever in Extended-Care Facilities," *New England Journal of Medicine* 300 (1979): 1246–1250.

20. R. Cogen, B. Patterson, S. Chavin, et al., "Surrogate Decision-Maker Preferences for Medical Care for Severely Demented Nursing Home Patients," *Archives of Internal Medicine* 152 (1992): 1885–1888.

21. R. Uhlmann, R. Pearlman, and C. Kevin, "Physicians' and Spouses' Prediction of Elderly Patients' Resuscitation Preferences," *Journal of Gerontology* 213 (1988): M115–121.

22. J. Hare, C. Pratt, and C. Nelson, "Agreement between Patients and Their Self-Selected Surrogates in Difficult Medical Decisions," *Archives of Internal Medicine* 157 (1992): 1049–1054.

23. L. Volicer, Y. Rheaume, J. Brown, K. Fabiszewski, and R. Brady, "Hospice Approach to the Treatment of Patients with Advanced Dementia of the Alzheimer Type," *Journal of the American Medical Association* 256 (1986): 2210–2213.

24. R. Cogen, B. Patterson, S. Chavin, et al. "Surrogate Decision-Maker Preferences for Medical Care of Severely Demented Nursing Home Patients," *Archives of Internal Medicine* 152 (1992): 1885–1888.

25. D. Luchins and P. Hanrahan, "What Is Appropriate Health Care for End-

Stage Dementia?" *Journal of the American Geriatrics Society* 41 (1993): 25–30.

26. E. Emanuel and L. Emanuel, "Proxy Decision Making for Incompetent Patients: An Ethical and Empirical Analysis," *Journal of the American Medical Association* 267 (1992): 2067–2071.

27. R. Brook and K. Lohr, "Monitoring Quality of Care in the Medicare Program: Two Proposed Systems," *Journal of the American Medical Association* 258 (1985): 338–341.

28. S. Mayer-Oakes, R. Oye, and B. Leak, "Predictors of Mortality in Older Patients Following Medical Intensive Care: The Importance of Functional Status," *Journal of the American Geriatrics Society* 39 (1991): 862–868.

29. K. Fabiszewski, B. Volicer, and L. Volicer, "Effect of Antibiotic Treatment on Outcome of Fevers in Institutionalized Alzheimer Patients," *Journal of the American Medical Association* 263 (1990): 3168–3172.

30. M. Gillick, N. Serrell, and L. Gillick, "Adverse Consequences of Hospitalization in the Elderly," *Social Science and Medicine* 16 (1982): 1033–1038.

31. J. Bamford, P. Sandercock, C. Waslow, and G. Muir, "Why Are Patients with Acute Stroke Admitted to Hospital?" *British Medical Journal* 292 (1986): 1369–1372.

32. J. Hill, J. Hampton, and J. Mitchell, "A Randomized Trial of Home-Versus-Hospital Management for Patients with Suspected Myocardial Infarction," *Lancet* 2 (1978): 837–841.

33. M. Spletter, *A Woman's Choice: New Options in the Treatment of Breast Cancer* (Boston: Beacon Press, 1982).

34. E. Loewy, "Treatment Decisions in the Mentally Impaired: Limiting But Not Abandoning Treatment," *New England Journal of Medicine* 317 (1987): 1465–1469.

35. M. Gillick, N. Serrell, and L. Gillick, "Adverse Consequences of Hospitalization in the Elderly," *Social Science and Medicine* 16 (1982): 1033–1038.

36. D. Doyle, A. Turpie, J. Hirsh, et al., "Adjusted Subcutaneous Heparin or Continuous Intravenous Heparin in Patients with Acute Deep Vein Thrombosis," *Annals of Internal Medicine* 107 (1987): 441–445.

37. T. Wetle, "The Social and Service Context of Geriatric Care," in J. Rowe and R. Besdine, *Geriatric Medicine*, 2nd ed. (Boston: Little, Brown, 1988), pp. 52–74.

38. U.S. Senate Special Committee on Aging, *Aging America: Trends and Projections* (Washington, D.C.: U.S. DHHS, 1988), p. 118.

39. P. Kemper and C. Murtaugh, "Lifetime Use of Nursing Home Care," *New England Journal of Medicine* 324 (1991): 595–600.
40. Hing, "Use of Nursing Homes by the Elderly."

2. Blessed with Vim and Vigor

1. U.S. Senate Special Committee on Aging, *Aging America: Trends and Projections* (Washington, D.C.: U.S. DHHS, 1988), p. 114.
2. V. Fuchs, "No Pain, No Gain: Perspectives on Cost Containment," *Journal of the American Medical Association* 269 (1993): 631–633.
3. D. Callahan, *Setting Limits: Medical Goals in an Aging Society* (New York: Simon and Schuster, 1987).
4. N. Daniels, "Justice between Age-Groups: Am I My Parents' Keeper?" *Milbank Memorial Fund Quarterly* 61 (1983): 489–522.
5. Callahan, *Setting Limits*.
6. J. Fitzgerald, P. Moore, and R. Dittus, "The Care of Elderly Patients with Hip Fracture: Changes since Implementation of the Prospective Payment System," *New England Journal of Medicine* 319 (1988): 1392–1397.
7. U.S. Department of HEW, *Vital Statistics of the United States, Vol. II—Mortality* (Washington, D.C.: U.S. Government Printing Office, 1982), Table 6-3.
8. J. Avorn, "Benefit and Cost Analysis in Geriatric Care: Turning Age Discrimination into Health Policy," *New England Journal of Medicine* 310 (1984): 1294–1301.
9. President's Commission for the Study of Ethical Problems in Medicine and Biomedical and Behavioral Research, *Making Health Care Decisions* (Washington, D.C.: U.S. Government Printing Office, 1982).
10. M. Gillick, "Common-sense Models of Health and Disease," *New England Journal of Medicine* 313 (1985): 700–703.
11. J. Katz, *The Silent World of Doctor and Patient* (New York: Free Press, 1984).
12. R. Blendon and D. Altmann, "Public Attitudes about Health-Care Costs: A Lesson in National Schizophrenia," *New England Journal of Medicine* 311 (1984): 613–616.
13. R. Butler, *Why Survive? Being Old in America* (New York: Harper and Row, 1975).
14. Callahan, *Setting Limits*.
15. President's Commission for the Study of Ethical Problems in Medicine and Biomedical and Behavioral Research, *Decisions to Forego Life-*

Sustaining Treatment (Washington, D.C.: U.S. Government Printing Office, 1982); L. Emanuel and E. Emanuel, "The Medical Directive: A New Comprehensive Care Document," *Journal of the American Medical Association* 261 (1989): 3288–3293.

16. D. Brock, "Death and Dying," in R. Veatch, ed., *Medical Ethics* (Boston: Jones and Bartlett, 1989), pp. 329–356.

17. J. Fries, "Age, Natural Death, and the Compression of Morbidity," *New England Journal of Medicine* 303 (1980): 130–135.

18. E. Schneider and J. Brody, "Aging, Natural Death, and the Compression of Morbidity: Another View," *New England Journal of Medicine* 309 (1983): 854–856.

19. U.S. Senate Special Committee on Aging, *Aging America.*

20. U.S. Congress, Office of Technology Assessment, *Life-Sustaining Technologies and the Elderly*, OTA-OA-306 (Washington, D.C.: U.S. Government Printing Office, 1987).

21. Ibid.

22. R. Nicholson, "Truth Lies Somewhere, If We Knew But Where," *Hastings Center Report* 23 (1993): 5.

23. H. Aaron and N. Schwartz, *The Painful Prescription: Rationing Hospital Care* (Washington, D.C.: The Brookings Institution, 1984).

24. U.S. Congress, Office of Technology Assessment, *Life-Sustaining Technologies.*

25. L. Westlie, A. Umen, S. Nestrud, et al., "Mortality, Morbidity and Life Satisfaction in the Very Old Dialysis Patient," *Transactions of the American Society for Artificial Internal Organs* 30 (1984): 21–30.

26. S. Neu and C. Kjellstrand, "Stopping Long-Term Dialysis: An Empirical Study of Withdrawal of Life-Supporting Treatment," *New England Journal of Medicine* 314 (1986): 14–20.

27. D. Muller and E. Topol, "Selection of Patients with Acute Myocardial Infarction for Thrombolytic Therapy," *Annals of Internal Medicine* 113 (1990): 949–960.

28. J. Gurwitz, R. Goldberg, and J. Gore, "Coronary Thrombolysis for the Elderly?" *Journal of the American Medical Association* 265 (1991): 1720–1723.

29. S. Gold, W. Wong, I. Schatz, and P. Blanchette, "Invasive Treatment for Coronary Artery Disease in the Elderly," *Archives of Internal Medicine* 151 (1991): 1085–1088.

30. L. Edmunds, L. Stephenson, R. Edie, and M. Ratcliffe, "Open-Heart Surgery in Octogenarians," *New England Journal of Medicine* 319 (1988): 131–136.

31. United States Department of Health and Human Services, *Your Medicare Handbook,* Publication No. HCFA-10050 (Washington, D.C.: U.S. Government Printing Office, 1985).

32. P. Appelbaum and T. Grisso, "Assessing Patients' Capacities to Consent to Treatment," *New England Journal of Medicine* 319 (1988): 1635–1638.

33. S. Mayer-Oakes, R. Oye, and B. Leak, "Predictors of Mortality in Older Patients Following Medical Intensive Care: The Importance of Functional Status," *Journal of the American Geriatrics Society* 39 (1991): 862–868.

34. D. Miller, D. Jahnigen, M. Gorbien, and L. Simbarti, "Cardiopulmonary Resuscitation: How Helpful?" *Archives of Internal Medicine* 152 (1992): 578–582.

3. Facing the Final Days

1. A. Otten, "Can't We Put My Mother to Sleep?" *Wall Street Journal,* June 5, 1985, p. 35.

2. G. Annas, "Physician-assisted Suicide: Michigan's Temporary Solution," *New England Journal of Medicine* 328 (1993): 1573–1576.

3. P. Ariès, *Western Attitudes toward Death* (Baltimore, Md.: Johns Hopkins University Press, 1974).

4. D. Callahan, *The Troubled Dream of Life: Living with Mortality* (New York: Simon and Schuster, 1993).

5. M. Mannes, *Last Rights* (New York: William Morrow, 1973).

6. J. Lubitz and R. Prihoda, "The Use and Costs of Medicare Services in the Last Two Years of Life," *Health Care Financing Review* 5 (1984): 117–131; J. Lubitz and G. Riley, "Trends in Medicare Payments in the Last Year of Life," *New England Journal of Medicine* 328 (1993): 1092–1096.

7. S. Abramowitz, "Pain, as a Matter of Policy," *New York Times,* October 24, 1989, p. 27.

8. W. Knaus, D. Wagner, and J. Lynn, "Short-Term Mortality Predictions for Critically Ill Hospitalized Adults: Science and Ethics," *Science* 254 (1991): 389–393.

9. R. Truog, A. Brett, and J. Frader, "The Problem with Futility," *New England Journal of Medicine* 326 (1992): 1560–1564.

10. A. Brett, "When Patients Request Specific Interventions: Defining the Limits of the Physician's Obligation," *New England Journal of Medicine* 315 (1986): 1347–1351.

11. D. Murphy, "Do-Not-Resuscitate Orders: Time for Reappraisal in Long-Term Care Institutions," *Journal of the American Medical Association* 260 (1988): 2098–2101.

12. L. Schneiderman, N. Jecker, and A. Jonsen, "Medical Futility: Its Meaning and Ethical Implications," *Annals of Internal Medicine* 112 (1990): 949–954.
13. M. Danis, D. Patrick, L. Southerland, and M. Green, "Patients' and Families' Preferences for Medical Intensive Care," *Journal of the American Medical Association* 260 (1988): 797–802.
14. M. Gillick, "Talking with Patients about Risk," *Journal of General Internal Medicine* 3 (1988): 166–170.
15. R. Weir and L. Gostin, "Decisions to Abate Life-Sustaining Treatment for Nonautonomous Patients," *Journal of the American Medical Association* 264 (1990): 1846–1853.
16. M. Gillick, "Limiting Medical Care: Physicians' Beliefs, Physicians' Behavior," *Journal of the American Geriatrics Society* 36 (1988): 747–752.
17. R. Misbin, "Physicians' Aid in Dying," *New England Journal of Medicine* 325 (1991): 1307–1311.
18. D. Brock, "Voluntary Active Euthanasia," *Hastings Center Report* (March/April 1992): 10–22.
19. J. Ruark, T. Raffin, and the Stanford University Medical Center Committee on Ethics, "Initiating and Withdrawing Life Support," *New England Journal of Medicine* 318 (1988): 25–30.
20. R. Blendon, U. Szalay, and R. Knox, "Should Physicians Aid Their Patients in Dying?" *Journal of the American Medical Association* 267 (1992): 2658–2662.
21. P. Singer and M. Siegler, "Euthanasia—A Critique," *New England Journal of Medicine* 322 (1990): 1881–1883.
22. M. De Wachter, "Euthanasia in the Netherlands," *Hastings Center Report* (March/April 1992): 23–30.
23. E. Cassell, "The Nature of Suffering and the Goals of Medicine," *New England Journal of Medicine* 306 (1982): 639–645.
24. A. Kleinman, *The Illness Narratives: Suffering, Healing, and the Human Condition* (New York: Basic Books, 1988).
25. I. Illich, *Medical Nemesis: The Expropriation of Health* (New York: Random House, 1976).
26. M. Gillick, N. Serrell, and L. Gillick, "Adverse Consequences of Hospitalization in the Elderly," *Social Science and Medicine* 16 (1982): 1033–1038.
27. S. Stoddard, *The Hospice Movement: A Better Way of Caring for the Dying* (New York: Random House, 1978).

28. J. Rhymes, "Hospice Care in America," *Journal of the American Medical Association* 264 (1990): 369–372.
29. W. Bulkin and H. Lukashok, "Rx for Dying: The Case for Hospice," *New England Journal of Medicine* 318 (1988): 376–378.
30. D. Greer and V. Mor, "How Medicare Is Altering the Hospice Movement," *Hastings Center Report* 15 (1985): 5–13.
31. R. Kane, L. Bernstein, J. Wales, et al., "A Randomised, Controlled Trial of Hospice Care," *Lancet* 1 (1984): 890–894.
32. National Center for Health Statistics, *Advance Report of Mortality Statistics, 1984,* Monthly Vital Statistics Report, vol. 35, no. 6, suppl. 2, September 1986.

4. Living with Limited Reserves

1. T. Quill, *Death and Dignity: Making Choices and Taking Charge* (New York: W. W. Norton, 1993); B. Friedan, *The Fountain of Age* (New York: Simon and Schuster, 1993).
2. J. Guralnik and E. Simonsick, "Physical Disability in Older Americans," *Journal of Gerontology* 48 (1993): 3–10.
3. M. Johnston and L. Miller, "Cost-Effectiveness of the Medicare Three-Hour Regulation,"*Archives of Physical Medicine and Rehabilitation* 67 (1986): 581–584.
4. R. Safian, A. Berman, D. Diver, et al., "Balloon Aortic Valvuloplasty in 170 Consecutive Patients," *New England Journal of Medicine* 319 (1988): 125–130.
5. L. Edmunds, L. Stephenson, and R. Edie, "Open Heart Surgery in Octogenarians," *New England Journal of Medicine* 319 (1988): 131–136.
6. A. Malcolm, "Giving Death a Hand: Rending Issue," *New York Times,* June 6, 1990, p. A6.
7. M. Creditor, "The Hazards of Hospitalization of the Elderly," *Annals of Internal Medicine* 118 (1993): 219–223.
8. *Vital Statistics of the United States: Expectation of Life at Single Years of Age, by Race and Sex* (Washington, D.C.: U.S. Government Printing Office, 1982), Table 6-3.
9. U.S. Senate Special Committee on Aging, *Aging America: Trends and Projections* (Washington, D.C.: U.S. Government Printing Office, 1988).
10. L. Verbrugge, "Longer Life but Worsening Health: Trends in Health and Mortality of Middle-Aged and Older Persons," *Milbank Memorial Fund Quarterly* 62 (1984): 475–519.

11. U.S. Senate Special Committee on Aging, *Aging America*, Table 4-2.
12. D. Evans, H. Funkenstein, M. Albert, et al., "Prevalence of Alzheimer's Disease in a Community Population of Older Persons," *Journal of the American Medical Association* 262 (1989): 2551–2556.
13. T. Wetle, "The Social and Service Context of Geriatric Care," in J. Rowe and R. Besdine, *Geriatric Medicine*, 2nd ed. (Boston: Little, Brown, 1988), pp. 52–74.
14. U.S. Senate Special Committee on Aging, *Aging America*.
15. Wetle, "The Social and Service Context of Geriatric Care."
16. S. Sheehan, *Kate Quinton's Days* (Boston: Houghton Mifflin, 1984).
17. M. Mendelsohn, *Tender Loving Greed* (New York: Alfred A. Knopf, 1974); B. Vladeck, *Unloving Care: The Nursing Home Tragedy* (New York: Basic Books, 1990).
18. M. Beers, J. Avorn, S. Soumerai, et al., "Psychoactive Medication Use in Intermediate Care Facility Residents," *Journal of the American Medical Association* 260 (1988): 3016–3020.
19. L. Libow and P. Starer, "Care of the Nursing Home Patient," *New England Journal of Medicine* 321 (1989): 93–96.
20. R. Kane and A. Caplan, *Everyday Ethics: Resolving Dilemmas in Nursing Home Life* (New York: Springer, 1990).
21. R. Ross and J. La Puma, "The Ethics of Mechanical Restraints," *Hastings Center Report* (January–February 1991): 22–25.
22. Institute of Medicine, *Improving the Quality of Care in Nursing Homes* (Washington, D.C.: National Academy Press, 1986).
23. C. Haber, *Beyond Sixty-Five: The Dilemma of Old Age in America's Past* (Cambridge: Cambridge University Press, 1983).
24. Ibid.
25. E. Emanuel, "A Review of the Ethical and Legal Aspects of Terminating Medical Care," *American Journal of Medicine* 84 (1988): 291–301.
26. R. Veatch, *Death, Dying, and the Biological Revolution: Our Last Quest for Responsibility,* rev. ed. (New Haven: Yale University Press, 1989).
27. R. Weir and L. Gostin, "Decisions to Abate Life-Sustaining Treatment for Nonautonomous Patients: Ethical Standards and Legal Liability for Physicians after Cruzan," *Journal of the American Medical Association* 264 (1990): 1846–1853.
28. C. Sprung, "Changing Attitudes and Practices in Forgoing Life-Sustaining Treatments," *Journal of the American Medical Association* 263 (1990): 2211–2215.
29. A. Brett, "When Patients Request Specific Interventions: Defining the

Limits of the Physician's Obligation," *New England Journal of Medicine* 315 (1986): 1347–1351.

30. J. Katz, *The Silent World of Doctor and Patient* (New York: The Free Press, 1984).
31. P. Appelbaum and T. Grisso, "Assessing Patients' Capacities to Consent to Treatment," *New England Journal of Medicine* 319 (1988): 1635–1638.
32. A. Buchanan and D. Brock, *Deciding for Others: The Ethics of Surrogate Decision Making* (Cambridge: Cambridge University Press, 1989).

5. The Means to the Ends

1. E. Kubler-Ross, *On Death and Dying* (New York: Macmillan, 1969).
2. M. Sager, D. Easterling, D. Kindig, and O. Anderson, "Changes in the Location of Death after the Passage of Medicare's Prospective Payment System," *New England Journal of Medicine* 320 (1989): 433–439.
3. R. Hoopes, "Working Late: The Railroad to Retirement—Tips on How to Avoid Being Kicked Out," *Modern Maturity*, February–March 1989.
4. A. Berman, "A Passion for Living," *Modern Maturity*, June–July 1989.
5. Letter to the Editor, *Modern Maturity*, June–July 1989, p. 7.
6. R. Earle and D. Imrie, *Your Vitality Quotient: The Clinically Proven Program That Can Reduce Your Body Age and Increase Your Zest for Life* (New York: Warner Books, 1990).
7. S. Berger, *Forever Young: 20 Years Younger in 20 Weeks: Dr. Berger's Step-by-Step Rejuvenating Program* (New York: Avon Books, 1990).
8. S. Miller, J. Miller, and D. Miller, *Conquest of Aging: The Definitive Home Medical Reference from a Panel of Distinguished Medical Authorities* (New York: Collier Books, 1986), p. 8.
9. Ibid., p. 2.
10. M. Fiatarone, E. Markis, N. Ryan, et al., "High-Intensity Strength Training in Nonagenarians: Effects on Skeletal Muscle," *Journal of the American Medical Association* 263 (1990): 3029–3034.
11. J. Rowe and R. Kahn, "Human Aging: Usual and Successful," *Science* 237 (1987): 143–149.
12. Miller, Miller, and Miller, *Conquest of Aging*, p. 146.
13. D. Selkoe, "Amyloid Protein and Alzheimer's Disease," *Scientific American* 265 (1991): 68–78.
14. K. Davis, L. Thal, E. Gamzu, et al., "A Double-Blind, Placebo-Controlled Multicenter Study of Tacrine for Alzheimer's Disease," *New England Journal of Medicine* 327 (1992): 1253–1259.

15. Miller, Miller, and Miller, *Conquest of Aging,* p. 157.
16. A. Jonsen and S. Toulmin, *The Abuse of Casuistry: A History of Moral Reasoning* (Berkeley: University of California Press, 1988); D. Davis, "Rich Cases: The Ethics of Thick Description," *Hastings Center Report* 21(4) (1991): 12–16.
17. R. Veatch, *Death, Dying, and the Biological Revolution* (New Haven: Yale University Press, 1989), p. 78.
18. M. Konner, *Medicine at the Crossroads* (New York: Pantheon, 1993).
19. E. Emanuel, *The Ends of Human Life: Medical Ethics in a Liberal Polity* (Cambridge, Mass.: Harvard University Press, 1991).
20. D. Callahan, *What Kind of Life: The Limits of Medical Progress* (New York: Simon and Schuster, 1990).
21. *Twenty-Third Annual Report of Charity of Massachusetts* (Boston: Wright and Potter, 1900).
22. Admission applications, Winchester Home for Aged Women. Archives, Schlesinger Library of Radcliffe College, Cambridge, Massachusetts.
23. R. A. Kane and R. L. Kane, *Long Term Care: Principles, Programs, and Policies* (New York: Springer, 1987).
24. M. Gillick, "The Role of the Rules: The Impact of the Bureaucratization of Long-Term Care," in R. Carson, K. Toombs, and D. Barnard, eds., *Chronic Illness: From Experience to Policy* (Bloomington: Indiana University Press, forthcoming).
25. P. Kemper and C. Murtaugh, "Lifetime Use of Nursing Home Care," *New England Journal of Medicine* 324 (1991): 595–600.
26. E. Goffman, *Asylums* (New York: Doubleday, 1961).
27. J. Avorn and E. Langer, "Induced Disability in Nursing Home Patients: A Controlled Trial," *Journal of the American Geriatrics Society* 30 (1982): 397–400.
28. H. Bursztajn, R. Feinbloom, R. Hamm, and A. Brodsky, *Medical Choices, Medical Chances: How Patients, Families, and Physicians Can Cope with Uncertainty* (New York: Routledge, 1990).
29. S. Greenfield, E. Nelson, M. Zubhoff, et al., "Variation in Resource Utilization among Medical Specialties and Systems of Care," *Journal of the American Medical Association* 267 (1992): 1624–1630.
30. B. Hillman, C. Joseph, M. Mabry, et al., "Frequency and Costs of Diagnostic Imaging in Office Practice: A Comparison of Self-Referring and Radiologist-Referring Physicians," *New England Journal of Medicine* 323 (1990): 1604–1608.
31. E. Saunders, E. Hickler, S. Hall, et al., "A Geriatric Special Care Unit:

Experience in a University Hospital," *Journal of the American Geriatrics Society* 31 (1983): 685–693.

32. J. Wennberg, J. Freeman, R. Shelton, and T. Bubolz, "Hospital Use and Mortality among Medicare Beneficiaries in Boston and New Haven," *New England Journal of Medicine* 321 (1989): 1168–1173.

33. D. Singer, P. Carr, A. Mulley, and G. Thibault, "Rationing Intensive Care: Physician Responses to a Resource Shortage," *New England Journal of Medicine* 209 (1983): 1155–1160.

34. K. Langwell and J. Hadley, "Capitation and the Medicare Program: History, Issues, and Evidence," *Health Care Financing Review,* Ann. Suppl. (1986): 9–19.

35. T. Rice and J. Gabel, "Protecting the Elderly against High Health Care Costs," *Health Affairs* 5 (1986): 5.

36. A. Somers, "Insurance for Long-Term Care: Some Definitions, Problems, and Guidelines for Action," *New England Journal of Medicine* 317 (1987): 23–29.

37. Health and Public Policy Committee, American College of Physicians, "Financing Long-Term Care," *Annals of Internal Medicine* 108 (1988): 279–288.

38. J. Ouslander, D. Osterweil, and J. Morley, *Medical Care in the Nursing Home* (New York: McGraw Hill, 1991).

39. Senate Select Committee on Aging, U.S. House of Representatives, *America's Elderly at Risk,* Publ. no. 99-508 (Washington, D.C.: U.S. Government Printing Office, 1985).

40. J. Keenan, J. Fanale, C. Ripsin, et al., "A Review of Federal Home Care Legislation," *Journal of the American Geriatrics Society* 38 (1990): 1041–1048.

41. J. Rhymes, "Hospice Care in America," *Journal of the American Medical Association* 264 (1990): 369–372.

42. Health and Public Policy Committee, American College of Physicians, "Financing Long-Term Care."

43. C. Harrington, C. Cassel, C. Estes, et al., "A National Long-term Care Program for the United States," *Journal of the American Medical Association* 266 (1991): 3023–3029.

44. R. Blendon, "The Public's View of the Future of Health Care," *Journal of the American Medical Association* 259 (1988): 3587–3593.

45. B. Lo, G. McLeod, and G. Sarka, "Patient Attitudes to Discussing Life-Sustaining Treatment," *Archives of Internal Medicine* 146 (1986): 1613–1615.

46. T. Finucane, J. Shumway, R. Powers, and R. D'Allessandri, "Planning with Elderly Outpatients for Contingencies of Severe Illness: A Survey and Clinical Trial," *Journal of General Internal Medicine* 3 (1988): 322–325.

47. J. LaPuma, D. Orentlicher, and R. Moss, "Advance Directives on Admission: Clinical Implications and Analysis of the Patient Self-Determination Act of 1990," *Journal of the American Medical Association* 266 (1991): 402–405.

48. M. Danis, L. Southerland, J. Garrett, et al., "A Prospective Study of Advance Directives for Life-Sustaining Care," *New England Journal of Medicine* 324 (1991): 882–888.

49. T. Fried, M. Stein, P. O'Sullivan, et al., "Limits of Patient Autonomy: Physician Attitudes and Practices Regarding Life-Sustaining Treatments and Euthanasia, *Archives of Internal Medicine* 153 (1993): 722–728.

50. J. LaPuma and E. Lawlor, "Quality-adjusted Life-Years," *Journal of the American Medical Association* 263 (1990): 2917–2925.

51. W. Roper, W. Winkenwerder, G. Hackbarth, and H. Krakauer, "Effectiveness in Health Care: An Initiative to Evaluate and Improve Medical Practice," *New England Journal of Medicine* 319 (1989): 1197–1202.

52. E. Brook, E. Park, M. Chassin, et al., "Predicting the Appropriate Use of Carotid Endarterectomy, Upper Gastrointestinal Endoscopy, and Coronary Angiography," *New England Journal of Medicine* 323 (1990): 113–117.

53. P. Dans, J. Weiner, and S. Otter, "Peer Review Organizations: Promises and Potential Pitfalls," *New England Journal of Medicine* 313 (1985): 1131–1137.

54. J. Lubitz and G. Riley, "Trends in Medicare Payments in the Last Year of Life," *New England Journal of Medicine* 328 (1993): 1092–1096.

55. Lo, McLeod, and Sarka, "Patient Attitudes to Discussing Life-sustaining Treatment."

Epilogue

1. J. F. Fitzgerald, P. S. Moore, and R. S. Dittus, "The Care of Elderly Patients with Hip Fracture: Changes since Implementation of the Prospective Payment System," *New England Journal of Medicine* 319 (1988): 1392–1397.

2. J. Lubitz and G. Riley, "Trends in Medicare Payments in the Last Year of Life," *New England Journal of Medicine* 328 (1993): 1092–1096.

3. D. Callahan, *Setting Limits* (New York: Simon and Schuster, 1987).

❖ *Index* ❖

Bones: broken, 49, 54, 55; hip, 183–184, 187; metastases, 189
Bowels, 4, 119
Brain: blood in, 17, 46, 61, 135, 139, 141; damage, 77; impaired functioning after surgery, 117
Brainwave tests, 135
Breast. *See* Cancer; Mastectomy
Breath and breathing: rapid, 29; shortness of, 37, 55, 61, 70, 94, 95, 99, 109, 115, 133, 134, 153, 182, 185; painful, 112. *See also* Oxygen; Respirators
Bronchitis, 107
Brophy, Paul, 141
Burnap Free Home for Aged Women, 158

Calcium channel blockers, 147
Calcium tests, 121–122
Cancer, 43, 103; abdominal, 3; metastatic, 3, 86, 103, 147, 185, 186; disclosure of diagnosis to patient, 23; breast, 34–35, 142, 147, 183, 185; intestinal, 54–55; rectal, 83–86
Carbon dioxide, 95, 96
Cardiac arrest, 26, 63, 68, 115
Cardiac catheterization, 175
Cardiomyopathy, 103
Cardiopulmonary resuscitation (CPR), 22, 26, 32, 79, 82, 154
Cardiovascular disease, 103. *See also* Heart
Caretakers: family, 24–25, 129; professional, 123–124, 152, 171
Cataracts, 4, 17, 183
Cathartics, 90, 102
Catheters: kidney, 61, 63, 65; arterial, 75, 110; bladder, 75, 111; brain, 175
Catholicism, 155
Chemotherapy, 3, 6, 68, 185, 186, 188, 189; side effects of, 187
Chest: pain, 55, 109, 110, 133, 134, 148, 182, 188; physical therapy, 95
Cholesterol, 180, 187
Cimetidine, 111
Circulation, 151. *See also* Blood
Cognitive function, 5, 6, 7, 8, 23
Colectomy, 67
Colitis, 113, 114, 117
Colon, 113

Coma, 22, 28, 140, 155
Comfort: vs. prolongation of life, 3, 83; as goal of medical treatment, 5–6, 12, 41, 48, 65, 83, 85–86, 87, 96, 103, 131, 136, 138, 139, 143–144, 154; maximization, 6; measures, 32; as goal of surgery, 56. *See also* Palliation
Computerized tomogram (CT), 3, 135
Confusion/disorientation: following surgery, 1, 56, 111, 117; in demented elderly, 35, 36; kidney failure as cause of, 60, 65; from medication, 90, 111, 118; from emphysema, 96, 99; from hospital environment, 101–102; in frail elderly, 105, 108, 121; from infections, 121
Conquest of Aging, 151–152
Constipation, 43, 86, 102
Cost/benefit analyses, 13, 50–51
Cost of health care, 8–9, 52, 152–154
Court cases. *See* Lawsuits, medical
Cramps, leg, 134
Crohn's disease, 119–120, 121, 123, 127
Cruzan, Nancy, 81, 137, 140
Curvature of the spine, 93

Day care, adult, 25, 123
Death: inevitability of, 4, 147, 149, 152–153; rates, 8, 34, 64; risk of, in treatment options, 66, 180; good death concept, 70, 101, 102; at home, 100, 149, 161
Decision making, 11–12, 180; by proxy, 2, 21, 26, 74–75; by patient, 6, 10, 27, 67–68, 117; flexibility, 13; by physician, 21, 154–155, 172–176; by family, 23–35, 51–52, 68; informed/informed consent, 27, 67, 106, 115, 117–118, 142; substituted judgment, 31; patient involvement in, 35, 43–44, 154; individual choice in, 154, 155–156. *See also* Surrogate decision making
Deep vein thrombophlebitis (DVT), 37, 38, 39–40
Dehydration, 28, 95, 105, 113
Demented elderly, 15–16, 22, 105, 150, 151, 152, 156, 157, 179, 189; statistics, 8, 9, 20, 40; defined, 11; treatment as torment, 16–24, 180; limited care for, 20, 21, 32; in nursing homes, 20, 21, 29, 31, 32, 34,